WHAT NURSES KNOW...

# P C O S

# WHAT NURSES KNOW...

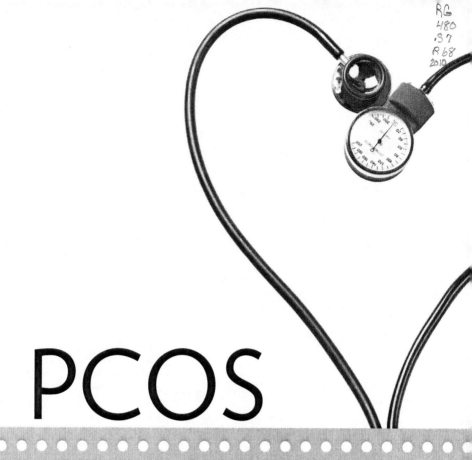

# PCOS

Karen Roush
RN, MSN, FNP, BC

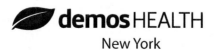

## demos HEALTH
New York

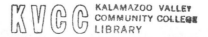

Visit our web site at www.demosmedpub.com

*Acquisitions Editor:* Noreen Henson
*Cover Design:* Steve Pisano
*Compositor:* NewGen North America
*Printer:* Hamilton Printing

Medical information provided by Demos Health, in the absence of a visit with a healthcare professional, must be considered as an educational service only. This book is not designed to replace a physician's independent judgment about the appropriateness or risks of a procedure or therapy for a given patient. Our purpose is to provide you with information that will help you make your own healthcare decisions.

The information and opinions provided here are believed to be accurate and sound, based on the best judgment available to the authors, editors, and publisher, but readers who fail to consult appropriate health authorities assume the risk of any injuries. The publisher is not responsible for errors or omissions. The editors and publisher welcome any reader to report to the publisher any discrepancies or inaccuracies noticed.

**Library of Congress Cataloging-in-Publication Data**
Roush, Karen.
    What nurses know-- PCOS / Karen Roush.
        p. cm.
    Includes index.
    ISBN 978-1-932603-84-2
    1. Polycystic ovary syndrome–Popular works. 2. Patient education. I. Title.
    RG480.S7R68 2010
    618.1'1–dc22

                                                            2009051276

Special discounts on bulk quantities of Demos Health books are available to corporations, professional associations, pharmaceutical companies, health care organizations, and other qualifying groups. For details, please contact:

Special Sales Department
Demos Medical Publishing
11 W. 42nd Street
New York, NY 10036
Phone: 800-532-8663 or 212-683-0072
Fax: 212-941-7842
E-mail: rsantana@demosmedpub.com
Made in the United States of America
    12 13          5 4 3 2

# Contents

# Foreword

Women living with polycystic ovary syndrome (PCOS) confront numerous questions about their diagnosis and treatment and often have a difficult time getting the answers they need. Realizing that something is wrong, but not knowing what, many women find themselves receiving a diagnosis in stages. Often they don't get a diagnosis of PCOS until after a number of other possibilities have been eliminated through testing and referral to yet another specialist. Management of PCOS has lifelong implications and can be as challenging as obtaining the initial diagnosis. Lifestyle changes and medications are basic to living well with PCOS. There *is* life after a diagnosis of PCOS. As the author of this volume suggests, you can learn to manage PCOS—it doesn't need to manage you.

This book is a valuable source of knowledge for women facing a diagnosis of PCOS and also for women who have lived with the condition for many years. The issues that women face, such as accepting their bodies, dealing with the potential health risks associated with PCOS, understanding some of the possible mental health consequences of life with PCOS, and the challenges of having children, can be overwhelming. This book is an outstanding source of information for any woman whose life is touched by PCOS, as well as family and friends who seek a better understanding of this condition.

This book is a wonderful resource that women living with PCOS will read and refer to again and again. It is a book that captures the wisdom amassed by a nurse whose practice undoubtedly has helped many women to live life well!

*—Nancy Fugate Woods, PhD, RN, FAAN*

# INTRODUCTION

# Living With Polycystic Ovarian Syndrome

I want to introduce you to two young women, both living with polycystic ovarian syndrome (PCOS). In some ways their stories are similar; in other ways they are dramatically different. This is not unusual in this most frustrating of disorders: there are many common characteristics, and yet PCOS can take many different shapes.

You'll be hearing from Stephanie and Amy throughout the book. If you are living with PCOS you will recognize their struggles and understand their frustrations. At times you will see yourself reflected in their words. You will know you are not alone out there. And you will know that you are not going crazy, you are not just lazy, and you are not less of a woman because of this disorder. Like Stephanie and Amy, you are strong, resilient, and brave. Like them, you feel tired and angry at times. And that is okay, because you have not given in to those emotions. If you had, you would not be reading this book. You persevere; you continue to pursue health and the best of life for yourself.

I hope this book helps you in that quest.

## How It Began

### STEPHANIE'S STORY

*The struggling with PCOS started about ten years ago, but I think it all really started when I was growing up. When I was nine years old I had torsion of the ovary and had to have major surgery. They left my ovary in and said everything would be normal. That's all I really know. A year later my mother died; she was killed by a drunk driver. I was too young to really know what was going on, so all the information about what happened was lost with her. And I've never had her to help with what I've been going through with this.*

*Things were pretty normal all through junior high and high school. I was average size, had normal periods. No extra hair or weight or anything like that. Then about ten years ago, when I was twenty-one or twenty-two, I started noticing I was gaining weight. I didn't think that much of it, thought it was because I wasn't as active as I had been in high school. So that went on for a couple of years, and then it was like I was exploding all of a sudden, just getting so fat.*

*Things just got so out of control so fast. I didn't have a period for one and a half or two years. I was married already, and even though we weren't using birth control I didn't get pregnant. At first I wasn't concerned; we weren't necessarily trying to have a baby. Then I started getting hair on my chin and my chest; that's when I realized something wasn't right.*

*I went to see an endocrinologist. She said I had PCOS and gave me Clomid. That's all I knew, nothing about what was happening to me. She was just into fertility and didn't tell me anything else.*

### AMY'S STORY

*I remember in high school my periods were really, really painful, so painful to the point that I had to stay home from school. I couldn't get out of bed. And I had no energy. No one knew what was going on; they checked me for mono and anemia and stuff. People said I was lazy. I wasn't lazy; I was so tired I couldn't even stay awake.*

*I was always overweight. My mom would get mad at me, saying I wasn't active enough, and make me go for bike rides or go rollerblading. I was on the field hockey team, and I was running as much as all the other girls on the team. I would do the same things they did at practice and then go home and run extra miles on the treadmill. Who wants to be the biggest, slowest one on the team? But I was, no matter what I did.*

*Then I started having really bad acne. I went to a dermatologist and he said I needed a blood test. No explanation why, just sent me for a blood test and gave me some acne cream to use. When he called my mom with the results her jaw dropped. She couldn't believe how incredibly out of whack my hormones were.*

*So next we went to an endocrinologist who did a whole bunch of blood tests. He asked me about my symptoms, and I told him about being tired all the time, having no energy, how I really didn't eat a lot and I was so much heavier than I should have been. He said, "I think you have PCOS," and sent me to an OB/GYN to get an ultrasound to look for polycystic ovaries. I had no idea what PCOS was. When the results came back, she said, "Yep, you definitely have it." It was right before my eighteenth birthday.*

# WHAT NURSES KNOW . . .
# P C O S

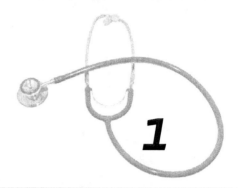

# What Is Happening and Why?

*The endocrinologist said, "You have PCOS. You're going to have to take these medications every day. You're going to have to live with this and deal with it through diet." That was it. I didn't understand what it was. Even now, it's hard to understand. There are so many things going on. It's this, this, and this causing this and this and this!   AMY*

**PCOS is a disorder of questions.** For those experiencing its symptoms it can seem as if no one really knows what's going on. Even the experts can't seem to agree on a definition. Just getting a diagnosis can be a challenge—often the first of many. Some women have to fight for tests to be performed; others feel as if their life is one round of never-ending tests. And answers may never seem…well, like answers.

Science hasn't yet come up with many of the answers to the questions of PCOS. The underlying cause is still unknown. The role of genetics is not well understood. The interactions between the reproductive system and the endocrine system are complex, so it's still unclear what causes what or where it all starts.

Another reason answers can be hard to come by is that the disorder has many different faces. There is no one right answer for everyone. Some women struggle primarily with reproductive issues; for others it's the metabolic problems or the physical signs, and for some it is every symptom that PCOS can throw at them. Coming up with best-practice recommendations across such a spectrum of presentations is a challenge: what is "best" for some women is not "best" for others.

**But there is good news.** We know much more today about the complex, interrelated hormonal and metabolic processes involved in PCOS, and this understanding is continuing to increase as a result of the considerable amount of PCOS-focused research taking place. More and better treatment options are available for the various symptoms. Attention is being paid to possible long-term effects of the disorder so that women with PCOS can enjoy good health throughout their life span. And health care providers know more about PCOS than they did in the past and are better prepared to manage women with the disorder.

Another positive development is the amount of information and support available to women with PCOS. There are numerous resources for women to turn to: support groups, online

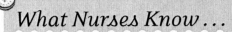

## What Nurses Know . . .

*As with any chronic condition, one of the most important things any woman with PCOS or PCOS-related symptoms can do is become an active participant in the management of her condition. This starts with getting the information she needs to ask the right questions and make informed decisions.*

chat rooms and newsletters, and books. Learning how to manage PCOS gives women back a sense of control over their life. Understanding what is happening is the first step on the path to managing PCOS instead of it managing you.

## What Is PCOS?

It was in 1935 that two doctors in Chicago, Irving Stein and Michael Leventhal, first described, in seven women, a group of symptoms that included amenorrhea (no periods), abnormal hair growth, infertility, and enlarged ovaries with multiple cysts. For many years these symptoms remained the hallmark of a condition that came to be known by many names: Stein–Leventhal syndrome, hyperandrogenic chronic anovulation, functional ovarian hyperandrogenism, and polycystic ovarian disease. Now it is most commonly called polycystic ovarian syndrome, or PCOS.

PCOS is a disorder found in women of childbearing age. The main features are menstrual irregularities and increased levels of androgens that can't be explained by other conditions. Women with PCOS often also present with infertility, insulin resistance, obesity, and polycystic ovaries. The type and severity of symptoms vary widely among women with the disorder.

Today PCOS is recognized as the most common endocrine disorder in women of reproductive age. It affects 5 to 10 percent of all women between puberty and menopause. It is the underlying cause of 90 percent of cases of infrequent menstruation and 30 percent of cases of amenorrhea. It accounts for 80 percent of cases of hirsutism (male-pattern hair growth in women).

Although the group of symptoms originally identified by Stein and Leventhal remains associated with PCOS, we now recognize that there's much more to the story. Until recently, PCOS was viewed as a disease of the reproductive system. Treatment focused almost exclusively on regulating the menstrual cycle and ensuring pregnancy. We now know that PCOS is also a metabolic disorder, and some experts believe that its metabolic component may be the central feature and hold the key to finding the cause of the disorder. (It should be called a disorder rather than disease)

## Definition of PCOS

Although it has been 75 years since Stein and Leventhal first described PCOS, there is still no international agreement on a definition. Three different sets of criteria for diagnosis have been proposed: the 1990 National Institutes of Health criteria, the 2003 Rotterdam criteria, and the 2006 Androgen Excess and PCOS Society criteria. These three sets of criteria are similar; the primary difference lies in whether they require polycystic ovaries to be present for a diagnosis of PCOS to be made.

It may seem odd that the principal disagreement is whether a condition called polycystic ovarian syndrome includes polycystic ovaries among its defining features. But polycystic ovaries

• • • • • • • • • • • • • • • • • • • • • • • • • • • •

## Definitions of PCOS

### The 1990 National Institutes of Health criteria
The 1990 National Institutes of Health criteria are the following:

- The presence of clinical hyperandrogenism and/or hyperandrogenemia
- The presence of oligo-ovulation
- The exclusion of related disorders

### The 2003 Rotterdam criteria
The 2003 Rotterdam criteria are the presence of two or more of the following, together with the exclusion of related disorders:

- Oligo-ovulation or anovulation
- Clinical and/or biochemical signs of hyperandrogenism
- Polycystic ovaries

### 2006 Androgen Excess and PCOS Society
The 2006 Androgen Excess and PCOS Society criteria are the following:

- The presence of hirsutism and/or hyperandrogenism
- The presence of oligo-ovulation and/or polycystic ovaries
- The exclusion of other androgen excess–related disorders

are found in up to 23 percent of women, of childbearing age and so there are many women who have polycystic ovaries but no symptoms of PCOS. There are also women with symptoms of PCOS who don't have polycystic ovaries. Therefore, many experts agree that a diagnosis of PCOS does not depend on the presence of polycystic ovaries.

Most people would agree that when something appears to be wrong, what they want most are answers. What is wrong with me? Why is this happening? When people have answers, when their condition has been named, they can move on to taking control of it and doing what they need to do to create the best life possible for themselves. Given all the questions surrounding the disorder and the lack of agreement on a definition, getting a diagnosis—naming what is going on—can be a frustrating process with PCOS.

Despite all the expert disagreement over criteria and which definition fits best, there is a bottom line: if you have any signs of too much androgen and fewer than eight or nine periods a year, and if no other cause can be found, you have PCOS.

Let's take a closer look at each of the criteria in the three competing definitions of PCOS.

### HYPERANDROGENISM AND HYPERANDROGENEMIA

Hyperandrogenism is characterized by the excessive secretion of androgens, primarily testosterone and androstenedione.

## Common Signs and Symptoms of PCOS

- Increased growth of coarse, dark facial and body hair
- Male-pattern baldness
- Moderate to severe acne
- Dark discoloration of the skin on the neck, thighs, and groin
- Skin tags
- Obesity
- Irregular periods or no periods
- Infertility

Androgens are commonly referred to as the male sex hormones because they are responsible for male characteristics and reproductive activity and because males make and use high levels of these hormones. However, females produce androgens as well, just in smaller amounts and for different purposes. (And, yes, males produce small amounts of estrogen.)

In females, androgens are produced by the ovaries, adrenal glands, and fat cells. They have a big role in a girl's transition to puberty. Throughout a woman's life they are important in the regulation of estrogen production, bone health, and sexual desire.

Clinical hyperandrogenism refers to the outward signs of excess androgens in women. In PCOS these signs include hirsutism (described below), male-pattern baldness, moderate to severe acne, and obesity.

It is important to note that although hyperandrogenism in PCOS causes hirsutism, male-pattern baldness, and moderate to severe acne, it does not cause virilization. Clinical signs of virilization—a deep voice, increased muscle mass, an increase in the size of the clitoris, or rapidly developing hirsutism or male-pattern baldness—point to higher levels of androgens than are normally seen in PCOS. If these signs are present, tests should be conducted to rule out ovarian or adrenal tumors.

Hyperandrogenemia is the presence of elevated levels of androgens in the blood.

### OLIGO-OVULATION AND ANOVULATION

Throughout their reproductive years, women usually ovulate once a month. Oligo-ovulation is irregular or infrequent

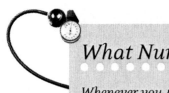

## What Nurses Know . . .

Whenever you see the suffix -emia, it refers to the blood.

ovulation (nine or fewer times a year). It results from mishaps in the complex hormonal signaling and feedback loops that regulate a woman's menstrual cycle.

Anovulation means that ovulation does not happen at all.

### HIRSUTISM

Hirsutism is increased hair growth on areas of a woman's body where it normally would be seen only in men, such as on the face, chest, and back. The hair is coarser and darker than usual. Hirsutism is the most common clinical sign of hyperandrogenism.

### POLYCYSTIC OVARIES

"Polycystic" means having multiple cysts (fluid-filled sacs). In PCOS, the ovarian cysts are follicles that started to mature but did not get to the point at which ovulation occurs, remaining in the ovaries as cysts.

## What Causes PCOS?

One of the reasons so many questions surround PCOS is that we don't yet know exactly what causes the disorder. A number of theories have gained support, but we do not have a full understanding of any of them.

### GENETICS

> *My mom probably had it. She died before all this started, so I never got a chance to talk to her about it. But she always struggled with her weight, and my dad said she had to take fertility drugs to get pregnant. So, yeah, I think she did have PCOS.*   STEPHANIE

PCOS runs in families. If your mother or sister has PCOS, you are five to six times more likely to have the disorder than other women. PCOS affects 35 to 40 percent of women who have an immediate family member with the disorder, compared with 5 to

10 percent of women in the general population. Although this indicates a genetic basis for PCOS, exactly how the inheritance works is unclear, and to date no genetic marker has been found. However, patterns of inheritance indicate that PCOS is an autosomal dominant disorder, meaning that a woman needs to inherit the defective gene from only one parent to develop the disorder.

Nevertheless, scientists aren't convinced that having one defective gene can fully explain PCOS. The enormous differences in how PCOS affects individual women suggest that multiple factors are involved. One theory is that a woman inherits a defective gene but that environmental factors determine how that gene affects her. Environmental factors can include diet, activity level, exposure to hormones (before and after birth), and events that happen when a girl is going through puberty.

There is also some evidence to suggest that it is perhaps not a single defective gene that causes PCOS but a combination of defective genes, each accounting for a separate symptom. When these genes occur together, a woman ends up with PCOS. Environmental factors are still thought to influence each individual's set of symptoms.

### ANDROGEN EXPOSURE

A second theory is that PCOS is caused by exposure to high levels of androgens in the uterus or at puberty. Androgens are steroid hormones that stimulate the development of masculine characteristics in a person. Scientists think this exposure can promote the symptoms of PCOS. However, we do not understand how this works. Evidence for this theory comes primarily from animal research showing that monkeys exposed to high levels of androgens in the uterus went on to develop many of the signs and symptoms of PCOS.

### INSULIN RESISTANCE

There is evidence that insulin resistance is not just one of the symptoms of PCOS but may be one of the underlying causes of the disorder. Insulin appears to have a number of roles in PCOS.

It increases androgen production in the ovaries and possibly in the adrenal glands, and it increases the amount of luteinizing hormone (LH) released by the pituitary gland. LH plays an important part in a woman's menstrual cycle (see below). Insulin may affect androgen production in women with PCOS as a result of a problem in the insulin signaling system. This signaling problem may result in high levels of insulin in the blood or in the ovaries being oversensitive to insulin in women with PCOS.

### OTHER POSSIBILITIES

PCOS has been found to be associated with low birth weight. One theory is that rapid catch-up growth in girls with low birth weight may promote excess levels of circulating insulin in the blood and increased adrenal gland androgen production.

PCOS has also been associated with epilepsy, although the underlying mechanism is unknown. Women with epilepsy have a much higher prevalence of PCOS than the general population: 11 to 26 percent, compared with 5 to 10 percent. It may be that changes in the brain that cause seizures also affect the release of hormones involved in PCOS. Finding the connection may help to explain underlying defects associated with PCOS.

## What Is Happening?

Understanding what is happening to your body will help you manage your symptoms and make informed decisions about testing, treatments, and lifestyle changes. It will enable you to be an active, engaged partner with your provider. You will know what questions to ask, and you will understand the answers.

You can refer to the glossary at the end of this book for the technical terms used. It is important to grasp the meanings of these terms so that you can "speak the language" of PCOS.

As is clear from the preceding section, we do not completely understand PCOS or what the underlying trigger is—or even whether there is one. But we do know that a number of abnormalities in hormonal and metabolic processes are involved and that they seem to be connected and to reinforce each other. After an overview of these hormonal and metabolic processes, we'll look specifically at what happens to hormonal control of the menstrual cycle in PCOS.

## HORMONAL AND METABOLIC PROCESSES

PCOS is an endocrine disorder: hormones, or your body's responses to hormones, are responsible for its symptoms. Hormones are chemical substances produced and secreted by specific glands or organs in your body that circulate via the blood to act on another part of the body. The glands and organs that secrete hormones make up the endocrine system. (Some organs outside the endocrine system also produce hormones, such as the kidneys and the heart, but hormone production is not their primary function.) Hormones have no activity of their own; their function is to regulate the activity of their target cells. Estrogen and testosterone are hormones. They regulate reproductive activity and the development of secondary sex characteristics. Insulin is also a hormone. It regulates the metabolism of carbohydrates.

**Understanding How Insulin Works.** Insulin is produced by cells in the pancreas; it helps move glucose from the blood into tissue cells, where it is used for energy. Insulin is secreted continuously in small amounts (known as the basal rate) that enable the body constantly to metabolize glucose for ongoing energy requirements. When the level of glucose in the blood rises after we eat, the pancreas responds by producing and secreting more insulin to metabolize the extra glucose. When the blood glucose level drops back to normal, secretion returns to the basal rate. This feedback loop maintains our blood glucose within the normal range necessary for optimal cell functioning.

When tissue cells do not respond to insulin adequately—when they resist the action of insulin—the result is a condition known as insulin resistance. In a person with insulin resistance, the glucose level in the blood is increased because cells aren't metabolizing glucose the way they should. The pancreas responds to the increased concentration of glucose by secreting more insulin, which results in hyperinsulinemia (too much insulin in the blood). It is not clear what causes insulin resistance in women with PCOS, but in the general population obesity, lack of exercise, a high-carbohydrate diet, and genetics are believed to be factors in the development of insulin resistance. Insulin resistance and the resulting high levels of insulin in your blood (called hyperinsulinemia) are believed to be key problems underlying PCOS.

**Insulin Resistance and PCOS.** Most women with PCOS have insulin resistance. This is true regardless of whether they are thin, of normal weight, or obese. There appears to be a type of insulin resistance that is inbuilt in women with PCOS. (Insulin resistance is more severe in obese women with PCOS, however, because they have an added degree of resistance secondary to their excess weight.)

Insulin resistance has a double whammy effect on androgen levels. Insulin works in cooperation with LH to increase androgen production by the ovaries, and it decreases the production of sex hormone–binding globulin (SHBG). SHBG binds with free testosterone in the blood, effectively removing it from the circulation, resulting in less testosterone being available to act on target tissues. Less SHBG means more testosterone. So the body's attempt to overcome insulin resistance—producing and secreting more insulin—results in more androgens for it to use.

But the interplay between insulin resistance and androgens doesn't end there. Increased androgen levels actually lead to insulin resistance. It's the old chicken-and-egg puzzle: which came first? Do high levels of androgens lead to insulin resistance, or does insulin resistance lead to high levels of androgens? Currently, most experts believe that hyperandrogenism does not cause insulin resistance but does contribute to it. **The bottom line is that hyperandrogenism and insulin resistance create a vicious cycle in women with PCOS that must be interrupted.**

## MENSTRUAL PROCESSES

*For so many years I would have normal periods, then nothing; then they would come back regular again. It was kind of a roller-coaster, never knowing when they would be normal, when they'd disappear. But for the last three years, nothing.* STEPHANIE

To understand what goes wrong with the menstrual cycle in PCOS, you first must understand how a normal menstrual cycle works.

The menstrual cycle is controlled by the secretion and withdrawal of hormones, primarily gonadotropin-releasing hormone (GnRH), follicle-stimulating hormone (FSH), LH, estrogen, and progesterone. These hormones are secreted and withdrawn via a negative feedback loop: when the level of a hormone increases to a certain point, a message is sent to the appropriate gland to slow down or stop secretion; when the level falls below a certain amount, another message goes out and secretion picks up again.

The whole process begins in the hypothalamus gland in the brain. The hypothalamus produces GnRH, which in turn stimulates the pituitary gland to secrete FSH and LH. FSH and LH then direct the ovaries to secrete estrogen and progesterone. The menstrual cycle has two phases: the follicular (proliferative) phase and the luteal (secretory) phase.

**Phase 1: Follicular Phase.** The menstrual cycle begins on the first day of a woman's period. At this time estrogen and progesterone levels are at their lowest, cuing the hypothalamus to secrete more GnRH, which signals the pituitary gland to secrete FSH and LH. This causes several follicles in the ovaries to begin to mature. Each follicle contains an egg. FSH levels then begin to decrease, allowing only a single follicle to continue to mature. The mature follicle produces estrogen, the concentration of which peaks on about the twelfth day of the cycle. Stimulated by the increasing level of estrogen, the lining of the uterus thickens and develops a richer blood supply. When the level of estrogen peaks, there is a surge in LH, which triggers the release of an egg (ovulation) within one to two days.

**Phase 2: Luteal Phase.** The cycle now enters the luteal, or premenstrual, phase, which typically lasts from day 14 until day 1 of the next period. Under the influence of LH the follicle develops into a corpus luteum. The corpus luteum secretes estrogen and increasing levels of progesterone, which enhances the thickening of the endometrium. This prepares the body to accept an embryo if conception takes place. If fertilization does not occur, the corpus luteum shrinks, estrogen and progesterone production decreases, and the drop in progesterone causes the lining of the uterus to slough off. The woman's period begins, and the whole process starts over again.

For most women this cycle lasts for 28 days, but a range of 25 to 35 days is considered normal. Bleeding lasts for an average of five days, with a normal range of three to seven days.

**So what happens in the menstrual cycle of someone with PCOS? Simply stated, the signals are all out of whack.** The feedback loop starts to misfire all the way back in the hypothalamus. An abnormally high frequency of GnRH secretion from the hypothalamus leads to higher than normal levels of LH and lower than normal levels of FSH. The lack of FSH means follicles don't mature, which means that ovulation does not take place. No ovulation means no progesterone production. The endometrium continues to thicken because of the high levels of estrogen, but there is no dropping progesterone level to trigger it to shed. Breakthrough bleeding may occur when the endometrium becomes too thick and superficial layers slough off, or if estrogen levels drop spontaneously. Lack of ovulation results in the reproductive system problems that women with PCOS experience: menstrual irregularities and infertility.

The challenges inherent in understanding and managing PCOS are now clear: all kinds of feedback loops and interactions are at work. Increased levels of LH and insulin increase androgen levels, which increases LH and insulin levels, which increases androgens. Increased androgen levels lead to insulin resistance, which leads to hyperandrogenism, which leads to increased insulin, which leads to increased androgens, which leads to...Increased body fat leads to insulin resistance, which leads to increased androgens, which leads to increased body fat, which leads to...

Stop! Do not be discouraged. There is one good thing about feedback loops: interrupt them anywhere and the cycle stops.

You can control PCOS. It's time to take back your life. The first step is getting a diagnosis.

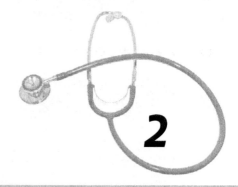

**2**

# Getting a Diagnosis

*I don't understand how they didn't know. Maybe if I had found out sooner I could have prevented some of it—having to go through all the weight gain and hair growth. Maybe I wouldn't have to struggle so much now. No one told me. No one checked for anything.   STEPHANIE*

Getting a diagnosis of PCOS can be challenging. No test gives a definitive diagnosis of PCOS; diagnosis is based on identifying a set of common symptoms and ruling out any other cause for them. A good diagnostic workup has three components: a thorough history, a physical exam, and laboratory and medical imaging tests.

## History

A diagnosis starts with a thorough medical, social, and family history. Your provider will ask you about current and past symptoms and their effect on your life. Some questions will be about common symptoms of PCOS, but many will not. Remember that one diagnostic criterion for PCOS is the exclusion of related disorders, so your provider will be looking for other possible causes of your symptoms, in a process called "differential diagnosis." When other causes have been ruled out, you and your provider can be more confident that PCOS is the correct diagnosis.

Many health care offices will send you a history form to fill out ahead of time; if they don't you can save valuable office visit time by preparing your own. (A sample history form is included at the end of this book.) If they do send you a form, make sure you're prepared to answer questions specifically related to PCOS that may not be on the form.

You can expect your provider to ask about the following key areas during the first office visit:

- General issues—fatigue, appetite, sleep problems (including snoring), sex drive

- Menstruation—first period, most recent period, frequency, characteristics of flow, pain and cramping, heavy bleeding
- Pregnancy—difficulty conceiving, surgery, number and outcomes of pregnancies, gestational diabetes, pregnancy-induced hypertension
- Body weight—problems with weight gain, dieting history
- Skin and hair—acne, hirsutism, male-pattern baldness
- Metabolic —diabetes, insulin resistance, glucose intolerance
- Cardiovascular system—hypertension, vascular disease, blood clots, cholesterol levels
- Cancer—personal or family history, abnormal Papanicolaou (Pap) smears
- Psychological issues—depression, anxiety
- Medications—what you have taken or are taking, what worked or didn't work, side effects
- Family history—issues in any of these key areas in your immediate family (parents and siblings)

## Physical Exam

The physical exam for PCOS looks for two things: signs of high levels of androgens and signs of other disorders that could explain your symptoms. The following sections outline the essential components of a physical to assess for PCOS; your provider may add other tests depending on your specific symptoms.

### BLOOD PRESSURE
High levels of androgens cause high blood pressure. Ideal blood pressure is lower than 120/80 mm Hg. If your blood pressure is between 120/80 and 139/89 mm Hg, you have prehypertension and you need to watch it. If your blood pressure is 140/90 mm Hg or higher, you should be treated for hypertension.

### HEIGHT AND WEIGHT
From your height and weight your provider can calculate your body mass index (BMI). BMI is a better indicator of body fat than

• • • • • • • • • • • • • • • • • • • • • • • • • • • •

## BMI

BMI = weight (lb) / [height (in)]2 x 703.
- Underweight: less than 18.5
- Normal weight: 18.5 to 24.9
- Overweight: 25.0 to 29.9
- Obese: 30.0 or greater

weight alone because it is a ratio of your weight to your height. A weight of 140 pounds on someone who is 5 feet 10 inches tall is very different from 140 pounds on someone who is 5 feet 3 inches tall.

### WAIST CIRCUMFERENCE

In PCOS any extra weight tends to concentrate around your middle. Your provider will measure your waist circumference, and may also take your hip measurement to calculate your waist-to-hip ratio. Because women with PCOS tend to have a larger waist circumference and waist-to-hip ratio they are at a higher risk for heart disease. For women, a waist circumference greater than 35 inches or a waist-to-hip ratio greater than 0.85 is considered to be a risk factor for heart disease.

### THYROID CHECK

The thyroid gland is located just below the larynx. For the exam, the provider will normally stand behind you, place the fingers of both hands gently on either side of your windpipe, and then ask you to swallow. The thyroid itself cannot usually be felt on exam; the provider is checking for any lumps or enlargement of the thyroid, as thyroid disease can cause many of the same symptoms as PCOS.

### SKIN EXAM

Your health provider will check for moderate to severe acne, skin tags (small harmless hanging pieces of extra skin) or acanthosis nigricans, a dark velvety discoloration of the skin usually seen in the folds of the neck, underarm area, or groin.

### HAIR EXAM
Your provider will look for signs of hirsutism or male-pattern baldness. Hirsutism is characterized by abnormally dark or coarse and excessive hair on the face or body. For accuracy your provider may use a chart known as the Ferriman-Gallwey score (explained in Chapter 6). Male-pattern baldness is characterized by a receding hairline on the sides of the head and thinning of the hair on the crown.

### PELVIC EXAM
A pelvic exam will be performed to assess the reproductive organs. Your provider may test for sexually transmitted infections or do a Pap smear for cervical cancer during the pelvic exam.

## Laboratory and Medical Imaging Tests

**No diagnostic test can tell you that you definitely have PCOS or that you definitely don't have it.** However, a number of tests can be used to evaluate your symptoms and to rule out other possible causes of them, leading to a diagnosis.

Providers take different approaches, and some will do more testing than others. Which tests they perform also depends on your particular set of symptoms. In your search for answers you may be thinking that you want all possible tests—that it can't hurt and maybe something will be discovered. However, there are good reasons not to rush into a lot of tests. Cost is one reason: some tests are expensive, and the money might be better spent elsewhere if the test is not going to help in diagnosis or management. More importantly, tests almost always involve some risk, and sometimes that risk can be significant.

Also, some tests carry a high chance of false-positive results. In other words, the test comes back saying there is something

## What Nurses Know . . .

If you are unsure whether a test is necessary, ask your provider two questions. First, do you need the test to decide on diagnosis or treatment and, second, will the results make any difference to how you manage your PCOS? If the answer to both questions is no, the test is probably not necessary.

wrong when there isn't, which can lead to unwarranted anxiety, needless follow-up testing, and even unnecessary treatment.

You will have blood tests, urine tests, and usually an ultrasound. If you are sexually active, you should also be given a pregnancy test.

Blood tests are used to check hormone levels, to look for signs of insulin resistance or diabetes, and to assess risks of cardiovascular disease.

*I constantly have abdominal pain or pressure. The endocrinologist showed me my ultrasound. Now I see why. My ovaries were huge and covered with follicles. She said they were chocolate chip cookie ovaries, and that's just what they looked like; there were so many follicles.   STEPHANIE*

A pelvic ultrasound can be used to check for cysts on the ovaries. However, polycystic ovaries are not always present in PCOS and are often present in women without PCOS, so a diagnosis of PCOS is not determined by whether you have polycystic ovaries, and not all providers will include an ultrasound in the diagnostic workup. You should discuss with your provider the necessity of this test. If you have pelvic pain or discomfort, bloating, breakthrough bleeding, or fewer than four periods in a year, you definitely should have an ultrasound. Magnetic resonance imaging (MRI) can also be used to look at the ovaries, but it is

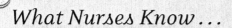

## *What Nurses Know . . .*

*Always follow up on test results. Do not assume that results must be normal if you don't hear anything. Test results can get lost, overlooked, or set aside in someone's busy day. When you have a test done ask how long it will take to get the results back, and if you don't hear from your provider within a day or two of that time, call them. No one wants to overlook a significant test result, and if it did indeed slip off the radar your provider will be glad for the reminder.*

not the preferred test and it is quite a bit more expensive than ultrasound.

### LABORATORY TESTS OF HORMONE LEVELS

This first group of tests looks at the levels of hormones that have a role in PCOS and its symptoms. (See Chapter 1 for a discussion of each hormone.) These hormone levels can vary greatly among women with PCOS and may even be normal in many cases, so these tests are used primarily to rule out other possible causes of PCOS symptoms. Be sure to mention to your provider whether you are taking any hormones or steroids as these can affect the results of many of these tests.

**Testosterone.** There are two types of testosterone tests: total testosterone and free testosterone. Total testosterone measures both the free and the bound testosterone in your blood. Bound testosterone is testosterone that is already bound to another molecule such as SHBG while free testosterone is freely circulating in the blood. The total testosterone level is more useful. In PCOS the total testosterone level may be normal or elevated. The main reason for doing this test is to rule out ovarian or adrenal tumors as the source of excess androgen. If the level is 200 ng/dL or higher, further testing for androgen-producing tumors is required.

This test is usually done in the morning, when testosterone levels are highest.

You can eat and drink before this test.

**Luteinizing Hormone/Follicle-Stimulating Hormone.**   It used to be routine to test LH and FSH levels, especially the LH-to-FSH ratio, and many providers continue to do so. However, even though we know that the frequency of LH secretion is increased in PCOS, up to a third of women with PCOS have normal LH levels. So the results of this test really don't help in making a definitive diagnosis.

You can eat and drink before this test.

**Dehydroepiandrosterone Sulfate.**   Dehydroepiandrosterone sulfate concentrations may be normal or slightly elevated in women with PCOS. If levels are 800 µg/dL or higher, testing for an adrenal tumor should be done.

You can eat and drink before this test.

**Prolactin.**   Prolactin, the hormone the controls lactation, is secreted by the pituitary gland. High levels can cause missed periods, so this test is included if that is one of your symptoms. PCOS can cause transient mildly elevated levels of prolactin. If elevated levels are found, then retesting is necessary because persistent elevated levels indicate the possibility of other causes. Very high levels of prolactin may indicate a pituitary tumor.

This test is performed in the morning.

You can eat and drink before this test

**Thyroid-Stimulating Hormone.**   A thyroid-stimulating hormone (TSH) test is done to rule out thyroid disease as a cause of menstrual irregularity or infertility. TSH controls the secretion of thyroid hormones. Abnormal results should be followed up for thyroid disease. Some controversy surrounds the optimum cutoff for the upper normal level of TSH, and you should talk to your provider if your level is above 2. (See Chapter 3 for more information on the treatment of thyroid disease in the context of PCOS.)

You can eat and drink before this test.

**Twenty-Four-Hour Urinary Free Cortisol.**   This test is used to rule out Cushing's syndrome as the cause of your symptoms. Your cortisol level may be slightly increased with PCOS, but levels twice as high as normal indicate Cushing's syndrome. Even mild elevations need follow-up evaluation for Cushing's.

You can eat and drink before this test.

**17-Hydroxyprogesterone.**   This blood test is performed to rule out late-onset congenital adrenal hyperplasia (CAH) as a cause of your symptoms. If you are taking birth control pills or steroids check with your provider about discontinuing them before having this test done.

### ADDITIONAL LABORATORY TESTS

The following tests are not diagnostic but are usually done at the same time as the diagnostic workup or shortly thereafter. They assess for disorders that often accompany PCOS, specifically insulin resistance, diabetes, and cardiovascular disease.

**Fasting Blood Sugar (FBS).**   This test measures the blood glucose concentration. It is usually carried out as part of the initial diagnosis and then repeated for ongoing evaluation of insulin resistance. An abnormally high result may indicate diabetes, insulin resistance, or glucose intolerance, and further testing should be done.

Blood is drawn after fasting for at least eight hours, usually first thing in the morning.

**Glucose Tolerance Test.**   This test measures how your body handles a normal amount of glucose over time. It is usually only done after you have been diagnosed with PCOS or if you have an abnormal fasting blood sugar.

A fasting blood sugar test is drawn first, and then you will drink a very sweet sugar solution. (This is not as tasty as it sounds; in fact, it sometimes causes nausea or sweating.) Blood is drawn to check the glucose level 30 minutes later and then every hour, for a total of four tests. Urine is collected every hour and checked to see whether you are "spilling" sugar into your urine. The result should be negative: no sugar in the urine.

You should not have anything to eat or drink except water for 12 hours before the test and during the test. You should not use tobacco products during the test as they can affect the results. After the final blood and urine samples have been collected you can eat and drink normally.

An abnormal result can indicate insulin resistance, diabetes, Cushing's syndrome, or kidney failure, or it may be due to the use of steroids or diuretics.

**Lipid Profile.** A lipid profile looks at the levels of the different types of cholesterol in the blood. The results are an accurate predictor of cardiovascular disease. The high levels of androgens

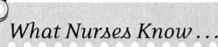

## What Nurses Know...

*"Normal" values represent what is considered the norm for most people, but not everyone will fall within the normal range. For many tests, results that fall slightly outside the normal range are not significant; for others, small differences in results can be very meaningful. Always review all abnormal results with your provider.*

*Also, what is considered a normal value for a blood test may vary slightly among labs. Keep this in mind if you are comparing results from recent tests with those from tests you have had in the past.*

associated with PCOS can result in abnormal lipid levels that increase the risk of cardiovascular disease.

You should not have anything to eat or drink except water for 12 to 14 hours before the test, which is usually performed first thing in the morning. Eating foods high in fat during the three to four weeks leading up to the test can affect the results.

### MEDICAL IMAGING

Pelvic ultrasound is the most commonly used medical imaging test in PCOS. An ultrasound provides information about the size of the ovaries (often enlarged in PCOS), the number and characteristics of follicles (cysts), and the thickness of the endo-metrium. A polycystic ovary is one that is increased in size (a volume of more than 10 cubic centimeters) or has 12 or more follicles measuring 2 to 9 millimeters in diameter.

Other medical imaging tests that can be used to look at the reproductive organs are MRI and a computerized tomography (CT or CAT) scan. These scans are much more expensive than a pelvic ultrasound and may require the injection of dye, which can carry a risk of side effects. These tests are required only if you have unusual symptoms or unexplained pain or there is sus-picion of a tumor.

**Pelvic Ultrasound.** Ultrasound tests use sound waves to visual-ize body structures. A transducer emits high-frequency sound waves that bounce off body structures back to the transducer. A computer connected to the transducer analyzes the signals and transforms them into two-dimensional images. All this happens in real time: the images are seen on the computer monitor dur-ing the test. No radiation is involved, and the test is considered risk free.

An ultrasound of the ovaries can be done from the outside, by moving the probe over your lower abdomen (transabdominal ultrasound), or it can be done from the inside, by inserting the probe into your vagina (transvaginal ultrasound). The preferred method in testing for PCOS is the transvaginal ultrasound because it gives a more accurate, clearer view of your ovaries, especially if you are obese.

A transvaginal ultrasound is not painful, but some women experience a little discomfort during the test because of the pressure of the probe. The transducer is shaped to fit into a woman's vagina and is smaller than the speculum used when you have a Pap smear. It is covered with a lubricated protective sheath, and only about two inches of the tip is inserted into the vagina.

A transvaginal ultrasound is not performed in young girls or in women who have never had sex involving penetration of the vagina. Of course, any woman has the right to refuse a transvaginal ultrasound and to have a transabdominal one instead.

A transabdominal ultrasound requires you to have a full bladder. Drink three or four glasses of water one hour before the test (about 10 ounces or 300 milliliters) and do not urinate until the test is over and the sonographer has conferred with the radiologist.

A transvaginal ultrasound does not require you to have a full bladder. If you are allergic to latex make sure you let the sonographer know so that a latex-free protective sheath is used on the transducer.

You can eat and drink before either of these tests.

## When It's Not PCOS

I've mentioned many times now that PCOS is a diagnosis of exclusion and that much of the diagnostic workup is meant to rule out other possible disorders as the cause of your symptoms. The following sections provide an overview of some of the more common possibilities your provider will be looking for.

### THYROID DISEASE

Problems with secretion of thyroid hormone can cause menstrual irregularities, hair loss, and weight gain. The most common cause is hypothyroidism, a disease in which insufficient thyroid hormone is produced. Women with hypothyroidism may also feel tired all the time.

### TUMORS OF THE OVARIES OR ADRENAL GLANDS

Tumors of the ovaries or adrenal glands can result in excessive secretion of androgens and menstrual irregularities.

### TUMORS OF THE PITUITARY GLAND

Tumors of the pituitary gland can cause problems with the secretion of LH and FSH, leading to irregular periods. They also cause hyperprolactinemia (see below).

### CUSHING'S SYNDROME

Overproduction of the adrenal steroid glucocorticoid can cause Cushing's syndrome as well as many of the symptoms seen in PCOS. Women with Cushing's syndrome have menstrual irregularities, obesity, hirsutism, and glucose intolerance or diabetes.

### CONGENITAL ADRENAL HYPERPLASIA

The rare classic form of this serious disorder is usually diagnosed early in a child's life; however, a mild form, known as late-onset CAH, can go undetected until puberty or later. In adults with CAH the adrenal glands do not produce enough of the hormone cortisol. This can result in an overproduction of androgens.

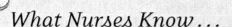

## What Nurses Know...

*Start a PCOS notebook. Keep a list of your medications and treatments and update it regularly. Include a section on diet and weight control and one on symptoms. Put copies of all your test results in the notebook. This way you will have an ongoing record that will help you see your progress and recognize any patterns that may have gone unnoticed. You can use the notebook to share information with different health care providers you see so that everyone is kept informed and up to date.*

Symptoms include menstrual irregularities, hirsutism, and infertility. Women with CAH may also have an enlarged clitoris, underdeveloped vaginal labia, frequent illnesses, and difficulty fighting off infections or healing from minor traumas.

### HYPERPROLACTINEMIA
Hyperprolactinemia is the presence of abnormally high levels of prolactin in the blood. It may cause menstrual irregularities as well as the spontaneous flow of breast milk. Hyperprolactinemia is often caused by a pituitary tumor.

Getting a diagnosis answers that first big question, What is this? Now it's time to answer the second one, What do I do about it?

## Resources

### Agency for Healthcare Research and Quality
Has a helpful resource about medical tests: "Quick Tips—When Getting Medical Tests."
www.ahrq.gov/consumer/quicktips/tiptests.htm

### Lab Tests Online
A Web site with a wealth of information about medical laboratory testing for health care consumers. PCOS is listed in the "Conditions/Diseases" box on the homepage.
www.labtestsonline.org/

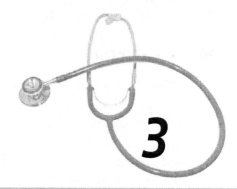

# Management of PCOS: The Basics

*The first endocrinologist didn't explain anything. Just said you're going to have to take these medications this many times a day. It felt like just take these medications and everything will be okay. I had no idea about insulin resistance. I didn't know to watch my sugar and carb intake. I admit I wasn't as good as I should have been about taking the medication, but I didn't understand the consequences either. Sometimes when I ran out of meds I wouldn't refill them right away and I didn't watch what I ate or exercise like I should have.   AMY*

*The doctor just wanted to start me on Clomid. I wasn't even trying to get pregnant then. I just wanted to get control of the situation so I could feel better mentally and physically. I was young and I felt so overwhelmed.   STEPHANIE*

So, you've gotten a diagnosis of PCOS. Now what? By now you won't be surprised to learn that there is no single answer to that question. Treatment for PCOS is not one size fits all. Your treatment will depend on your particular set of symptoms and how they affect your quality of life. It will depend on whether you're trying to get pregnant. It will depend on your risk for long-term problems such as heart disease.

Treatment for PCOS addresses five areas: regulation of your menstrual cycle, control of clinical signs of high levels of androgens, treatment of fertility, management of insulin resistance, and prevention of long-term risks. This chapter deals with the general approach to the management of PCOS. It discusses how to use what you've learned to be an active participant in managing your health. Detailed information on each type of treatment is provided in later chapters.

## Choosing a Provider

Should you see a specialist for PCOS, and, if so, what kind of specialist? Is it better to see someone who specializes in women's health or someone who specializes in endocrine disorders?

> The hardest thing was finding a doctor who actually cares about this, who will spend the time and explain things. It seems like there's just not enough knowledge out there, even with doctors. I finally found someone who paid more attention to me. Even though she was a reproductive endocrinologist she was more concerned with my overall health than just trying to get pregnant.   STEPHANIE

> Trying to find a good endocrinologist—that's the problem! How do you even know who's a good one? I really like my regular doctor but he doesn't really know enough about PCOS.   AMY

Initially it is best to see an endocrinologist, a doctor who specializes in problems with the body's hormonal system. **An endocrinologist is best equipped to guide you through the complex diagnostic workup and then work with you to design the optimum**

**management plan.** Subsequent management may require more of a team approach. Your goals and priorities will determine who makes up the team, and the team may change as your needs change. The team may include an endocrinologist and women's health provider as well as a general practitioner. If you are having difficulty getting pregnant, then a fertility specialist, usually a reproductive endocrinologist, needs to be added. Other health care personnel such as a nutritionist or dermatologist may join your team only for as long as they are needed.

Make sure that someone is keeping an eye on the big picture. Specialists focus on their specialty and may overlook issues that fall outside of it, one provider may order tests another has already done, and multiple providers can mean multiple medications that result in drug interactions or an overdose.

You need a coordinator, and often the best person for that role is a general practitioner, whose "specialty" is looking at the overall picture. Once you have a diagnosis and a plan that is working for you, your general practitioner can manage your ongoing care. He or she should keep other members of your team informed and seek their input.

During their reproductive years many women use their obstetrician/gynecologist (OB/GYN) as their primary care provider. Your OB/GYN may be in the perfect position to address the menstrual and reproductive system aspects of PCOS; however, long-term health effects such as an increased risk of heart disease and cancer also need attention.

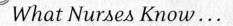

## What Nurses Know . . .

**Engage experts when you need to.** Severe acne may call for the expertise of a dermatologist. If you have anxiety or depression you may benefit from seeing a counselor. A nutritionist can help you design an optimum weight-loss diet.

## What Nurses Know...

*Every member of your team needs to be someone you trust and respect. You want people who will listen to your concerns, answer your questions, and be willing to work with other team members. PCOS is a complex, lifelong condition—choose people you'll want with you for the long haul.*

There is no hard-and-fast rule, but if you have multiple providers you must make sure they are all communicating with each other. At each visit ask the provider to send a record of the visit to other providers who are actively involved in your care.

### Overall Management Strategies: What You Can Expect

After diagnosis, you and your provider will decide how to manage your care. Make sure that the things that are important to you take priority. Perhaps your priority is hirsutism or weight gain. Perhaps it is irregular periods or infertility. You need to

## What Nurses Know...

*"Best practice" is an expression you will hear a lot when health care is being discussed. It refers to actions and treatments that are considered best for a particular condition or disease on the basis of the currently available evidence. Best practices are seen as the standard of practice—the acceptable and expected course of action to take. That doesn't mean they should always be applied to everyone. You and your provider should use best practices as a guide to figure out what is best for you.*

work with your provider to tailor management to your lifestyle and your goals. A plan based on best practice is only best practice if it actually works for you in real life.

Use your PCOS notebook to write down questions that come up between office visits. If you read or see something about PCOS write it down or put a copy into the notebook so that you can discuss it with your provider at the next visit. Keep an up-to-date list of the medications you're taking so that you can share it with each of the providers you see. Take the notebook to office visits and write down what you and your provider talk about, especially any instructions regarding treatments and medications. Schedule your next follow-up appointment before you leave and write the date and time in the notebook.

## Treatment Options

### Mainstays of PCOS Treatment

**Lifestyle changes**
- Weight loss
- Diet
- Exercise

**Hormonal treatments**
- Oral contraceptive pills (OCPs)
- Antiandrogens

**Insulin-sensitizing agents**
- Metformin

**Fertility treatments**
- Clomid
- Gonadotropins
- In vitro fertilization

**Skin and hair treatments**
- Excess hair removal
  - Mechanical removal
  - Medications
- Acne treatments
  - Skin medications
  - Oral medications
- Alopecia treatments
  - Scalp preparations
  - Oral medications

### SURGERY

For many years the recommended treatment for PCOS was an ovarian wedge resection, an operation to remove a large part of the ovary. The procedure had a good success rate; most women started having regular periods after the surgery, and many became pregnant. Unfortunately, it could also leave bands of scar tissue that prevented conception or increased the risk of a tubal pregnancy, a life-threatening condition in which the fertilized egg does not reach the uterus but begins to develop in the fallopian tube. Ovarian wedge resection is no longer recommended, but some providers continue to offer it as a treatment option. If your provider suggests this, you should ask why he or she thinks it's the best course for you despite newer, less risky options such as laparoscopic ovarian drilling, which uses either laser treatment or electrocoagulation to drill multiple small holes in each ovary.

Either of these surgeries is a last option for the treatment of infertility and is usually performed only when other treatments have failed. It is wise to get a second opinion before proceeding with any elective surgery. (For more information on these procedures, see Chapter 9).

### COMPLEMENTARY AND ALTERNATIVE THERAPIES

You will hear or read about "natural" therapies for PCOS. These are therapies that fall under the general heading of "complementary and alternative medicine" (CAM). They include herbal medicine, dietary supplements, acupuncture, naturopathy, and biofeedback. Complementary therapies are those that are combined with standard treatments, while alternative treatments are those used in place of standard treatments.

One problem with most CAM therapies is that there is little scientific evidence that they work. Either they have not been studied or the available studies are too small to yield accurate, dependable information. Studies not only tell us whether something works; they also reveal possible harmful effects. When you use untested treatments you don't know what the risks are. You also don't know whether they will cause problems when combined with other treatments—whether standard treatments or other CAM therapies.

Another consideration is that alternative medications and dietary supplements are not approved or regulated by the U.S.

Food and Drug Administration (FDA). This means that there is no control over what the labels say, what quality control measures are in place, or how dosage consistency is assured.

Alternative, "natural" products are often promoted as being better than putting chemicals (in the form of drugs) into your body. Many people say that these products are less disruptive to your body's natural processes. Think twice, however, before spending a lot of money on an array of natural products. We know that lifestyle changes related to diet and exercise (which really are a natural therapy) are the best way to manage PCOS symptoms. We also know that certain medications are very successful in treating PCOS symptoms and preventing long-term complications. We cannot say the same for natural products. There is no reason to believe that using natural products is better than simply following the lifestyle recommendations discussed in the next chapter and taking well-tested medications when needed.

Nevertheless, some CAM therapies can be helpful when used the right way. CAM therapies include deep breathing, meditation, massage, and yoga—all activities that are safe and effective ways to decrease stress and increase your sense of well-being.

Studies suggest that some dietary supplements are helpful for women with PCOS. A daily multivitamin that contains vitamins A, D, and E as well as magnesium, calcium, boron, chromium, and zinc may be beneficial as it has been shown that it is important for women with PCOS to maintain adequate levels of these vitamins and minerals. Other potentially beneficial supplements for women with PCOS include saw palmetto for the treat-

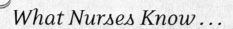

## What Nurses Know...

*There is no cure for PCOS. Do not trust any product or therapy that claims to be one.*

ment of hirsutism, garlic for its effect on blood glucose and blood pressure, and cinnamon for its effect on blood glucose.

When you are considering CAM therapy, you should take certain actions to decrease potential harmful effects and enhance potential benefits:

- Talk to your provider about the therapy and go over possible interactions with medications you are already taking.
- If you are trying to get pregnant be aware that some dietary supplements can decrease the effectiveness of fertility treatments and may be harmful to a developing fetus.
- Find information about the therapy through the Internet, articles, and books. Review the information you find with your provider. (See the resource list at the end of this chapter for a good Web site with information on CAM.)
- Talk to other women with PCOS who have tried the therapy.

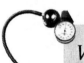

## What Nurses Know . . .

**Not all information is good information.** *A lot of information on the Internet is inaccurate, outdated, or biased. Pay attention to the organization the information is coming from. Is it an educational institution, government agency, nonprofit organization, or for-profit business? If products are recommended take a second look to see whether the Web site was developed by the company producing those products. Is the Web site really just a vehicle to promote a product, book, or service? What are the credentials of the person writing the information? When was the information last updated? The lists of resources at the end of each chapter includes trustworthy Web sites.*

● Avoid treatments that are available only from outside the United States. Other countries have different standards for quality and safety control.

## Follow-Up: How Much, How Often?

How often you follow up with your provider will depend on your response to treatment. If you are responding well, have no side effects from the medications you're on, and have no unusual or new symptoms, then an annual checkup with your primary care provider is usually enough. Blood tests to check your fasting blood sugar and lipids, a pelvic exam, and a Pap smear should be done. If you're on certain medications you may need additional blood tests (see Chapter 5). Of course, if your symptoms aren't getting better with treatment or there are any problems you will need to see your provider more frequently or follow up with the endocrinologist.

## Resources

### American Association of Clinical Endocrinologists
An organization of physicians specializing in endocrinology. Offers a search tool, Physician Finder, that will list endocrinologists practicing in your area.
www.aace.com/org/ (home page)
www.aace.com/resources/memsearch.php (Physician Finder)

●  ●  ●  ●  ●  ●  ●  ●  ●  ●  ●  ●  ●  ●  ●  ●  ●  ●  ●  ●  ●  ●  ●  ●  ●

## Follow-Up

You should follow up with the endocrinologist whenever you find yourself in one of the following situations:

● You are not responding to treatment or the response is not satisfactory.
● You exhibit signs of glucose intolerance or diabetes.
● You have rapid onset or worsening of hirsutism, male-pattern baldness, acne, or weight gain.

**National Center for Complementary and Alternative Medicine, National Institutes of Health**
This government-sponsored site provides research-based information on CAM for professionals and consumers. It covers an extensive list of treatments under the section, Topics A-Z.
http://nccam.nih.gov/

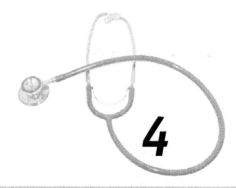

# Lifestyle Changes

*For years I didn't have a clue about what PCOS is. I started reading books and looking online. Now I'm more aware of what I have to do. I'm paying attention to what I eat. I haven't lost weight yet but I definitely feel better.   AMY*

*My advice to other women with PCOS? The lifestyle changes absolutely one hundred percent suppress symptoms. The hair growth is less and my sugar levels went down to normal.   STEPHANIE*

Lifestyle changes are the foundation of PCOS management. Most women who have mild to moderate symptoms should try weight loss, dietary measures, and exercise before starting on medications or fertility treatments. These lifestyle measures have been proven to improve symptoms associated with PCOS. If you are taking medications already, these measures will increase their effectiveness and may eventually lead to the medications being unnecessary.

## Weight Loss

If you are among the 50 to 70 percent of women with PCOS who are overweight, nothing you can do will bring as many positive effects as losing weight. And it doesn't take much: **losing as little as 5 to 7 percent of your body weight can lessen many of the symptoms of PCOS.** Weight loss will decrease testosterone levels and improve the regularity of your menstrual cycle. It will decrease insulin resistance and lower your long-term risk for cardiovascular disease and diabetes. As a result of its effects on androgen levels and ovulation, weight loss will also increase your chances of getting pregnant if you're trying to have a baby. And all of this without any of the potential side effects of medication.

> *My endocrinologist told me she wanted me to lose weight before we did anything else. I said I'd lose 25 pounds and call her. I lost 40 pounds! It cut my symptoms almost in half.* STEPHANIE

That said, losing weight isn't easy, and there is some evidence that for women with PCOS it's even more difficult than for others. Many women with PCOS have a higher than normal level of insulin in their blood, and insulin promotes the storage of fat. Remember that vicious cycle of PCOS? Increased body fat contributes to insulin resistance, which leads to increased weight, which increases insulin resistance, which contributes...well, you get the picture.

Science has discovered a lot about weight loss and obesity in the past 10 years. It is not just how much you eat that determines your weight; many people who are overweight metabolize calories and use energy differently than other people. We know now that hormones have a major role in appetite regulation. Research shows that people who are obese have problems with the actions of the two major hormones that affect appetite, ghrelin and leptin. Research also suggests that these problems are greater in women with PCOS than those without PCOS.

This doesn't mean, however, that you are destined to be overweight. There are measures you can take that will help you lose weight and keep it off despite your body's apparent determination to do otherwise.

The following section surveys weight-control advice based on the latest research. We talk about weight *control* because success is not just taking weight off; it's also keeping it off. But it's important to understand that the fact something works in a study doesn't guarantee it's going to work for you and your real life. And vice versa. So use these strategies as guidelines, talk to your provider, and keep trying.

### WEIGHT-CONTROL STRATEGIES
In weight-loss studies, four strategies are consistently associated with successful long-term weight control.

**Eating a Low-Calorie, Low-Fat Diet.**   There are all kinds of diets out there based on lowering caloric intake, eliminating certain foods, or eating a carefully combined set of carbohydrates, protein, and fats. Each of these diets has its avid supporters. Studies have produced somewhat mixed results regarding the best combination of carbohydrates, protein, and fats for weight loss, but whatever type of diet you choose, all studies agree on one thing: **it is the decrease in calories, not the composition of the diet, that leads to weight loss in all of them.**

The diet that most often comes out on top is a low-calorie, low-fat diet that consists of about 1,200 to 1,500 calories a day, with

## What Nurses Know...

*For your weight-control plan to succeed, it has to fit **your lifestyle**, it has to build on **your strengths**, and it has to overcome **your weaknesses**.*

no more than 30 percent of them coming from fat. Once you reach your ideal body weight you can increase your intake of calories to a level that allows you to maintain your weight while keeping your fat intake at 30 percent. Online calorie calculators can help you figure out your daily calorie needs, but make sure you use one from a reliable source, such as MayoClinic.com or WebMD.com.

You may be tempted to try a more extreme approach to lose weight faster, but studies suggest that this is not a good idea. Diets with extreme limits on fats, carbohydrates, or proteins—such as high-fat, no-carbohydrates or very-low-fat diets—are difficult to follow and can deprive the body of vital nutrients. Very-low-calorie diets (800 or fewer calories a day) have high dropout rates and high costs, and most people end up gaining back at least 50 percent of the weight they have lost. These diets may work in select cases for a short period but only under the close supervision of a medical provider.

**Eating Regular Meals.**    It turns out your mother was right about breakfast: eating regular meals spaced throughout the day has been shown to increase weight loss, and people who regularly eat breakfast are more likely to maintain their weight loss than people who don't.

**Maintaining a Consistent Diet 7 Days a Week, 52 Weeks a Year.**    Some people think that allowing themselves treats on weekends or holidays will relieve food cravings and help them stay on track over the long term. Studies show the opposite: giving yourself permission to eat badly on weekends or holidays can weaken your self-control and start you falling back into bad eating habits. Research has repeatedly shown that women who persist with healthy eating habits lose more weight and keep it off for longer than women who don't. This doesn't mean you can't indulge in the occasional treat; in fact, some flexibility in your diet has been linked with long-term success. No one can maintain rigid self-denial forever, and those who try to do so are more likely sooner or later to lose control and overeat.

**Self-Monitoring Body Weight and Food Intake Regularly.** Studies show that checking your weight regularly and keeping records of food intake promotes long-term success in weight control. When you keep a record of what you eat, how much you eat, and when you eat it, eating becomes a conscious, thought-out process. You pay attention to your food intake and the decisions you make about food.

In addition to these four strategies a number of others have been shown to be associated with successful weight control.

**Engaging in High Levels of Physical Activity.** High levels of physical activity increase weight loss and help keep weight off. Studies on the strategies used by people who have successfully lost weight and maintained their weight loss have found that almost all of them have used a combination of dieting and increased activity.

Exercise aids weight control through the calories you burn while doing the activity and through improved physical fitness, which lets you increase the intensity level of your activity over time and burn more calories. Studies have reported mixed results on the effect of exercise on appetite; some have shown that it increases appetite, others that it decreases appetite, and still others that it has no effect at all. (More information on exercise in relation to PCOS can be found later in this chapter.)

**Getting Support.** Support from your family and friends will help you stay on track with your weight-control plan. There is strong evidence that the support of family and friends enhances long-term weight control. The data for spousal and partner support are not so straightforward; sometimes it helps, sometimes it makes no difference, and in some studies partners were a bad influence.

When a couple are trying to lose weight together the mutual support can be very helpful. It can be difficult, however, for a partner to be supportive over time if they find *their* food choices being restricted by changes in *your* diet. It is a good idea to get your partner to buy into some of the dietary changes you're making;

after all, low-fat diets are recommended for everyone, whether they need to lose weight or not. Your partner can have larger portions of the same food you're eating and indulge in treats outside of the house. If they really want that ice cream after dinner, ask them to pick a flavor you don't like.

Ongoing support from professionals such as nutritionists, therapists, or your health care provider is also effective in maintaining weight loss. Having regular in-person meetings, even if they are as infrequent as every two months, results in greater weight loss and an increased likelihood that you'll keep the weight off. Phone contact has also been shown to be helpful—though not as helpful as in-person support. Some early studies suggested that Internet support programs might be helpful, but more recent studies have found that they are not helpful for the long term. Contact with a "real" person seems to be key in support programs.

What about formal weight-loss programs? Many people use commercial or professional programs and do very well with them. Weight Watchers is the only such program that has been studied scientifically, and the research shows it to be successful. Most people who succeed in losing weight on any program state that it is the weekly meetings that make a difference. Having to show up and answer to a group of fellow weight losers for what you ate all week and the change in your weight helps many people stay on track.

**Preventing Small Gains From Becoming Big Ones.**   If you do slip back into bad eating habits and start gaining weight, the less weight you allow yourself to regain, the less likely you are to go into a full relapse. It's not the small slipups that do you in; it's letting slipups become your normal eating habits again. Get right back on track each and every time and you'll be successful in the long term.

### WEIGHT-LOSS DRUGS

Drugs do not have a big place in weight-control strategies. First, any medication carries the risk of side effects, and, second, the benefits of weight-loss drugs are limited. Their effect lasts only as long as you are taking them, and usually you will gain back the weight when you stop. You cannot stay on weight-loss drugs forever. They have been tested for safety only for up to two years' use, and they normally lose their effectiveness after about six months of use anyway. **The safety of taking weight-loss drugs during pregnancy is not known, so you should not take them if you are pregnant or trying to get pregnant. They should also not be used if you are breastfeeding.**

That said, there are situations in which weight-loss drugs can be helpful—primarily if your BMI is above 27 and you have been unsuccessful in previous attempts to lose weight. Their use should always be combined with weight-loss counseling that includes dietary changes and exercise. Your plan should be to use the drug to get your weight loss started while you make lifestyle changes that will enhance your chances of long-term success.

The two most commonly used weight-loss drugs approved by the FDA are sibutramine and orlistat. Sibutramine (Meridia) requires a prescription; orlistat is available in both prescription strength (Xenical) and over-the-counter strength (Alli). Metformin (Glucophage), an antidiabetes drug used frequently in the treatment of PCOS, has also been shown to enhance weight loss in women with PCOS. It is discussed in detail in the next chapter.

Sibutramine and orlistat work very differently. Sibutramine is similar to medications used to treat depression and anxiety known as selective serotonin reuptake inhibitors (SSRIs). It is believed to work by suppressing appetite and increasing

## What Nurses Know ...

*Avoid over-the-counter appetite suppressants and weight-loss aids. There is no evidence that they work, and many are actually dangerous.*

the amount of fat you burn. In clinical studies, people taking sibutramine lost an average of 10 pounds more than people taking a placebo. However, it can increase your heart rate, raise your blood pressure, and cause an irregular heartbeat. You should not take sibutramine if you have high blood pressure or any history of heart disease or if you are already taking an SSRI. You should be on reliable birth control if you are taking sibutramine. Though there are no studies conducted on the use of this drug in pregnant women, birth abnormalities were found in animal studies.

Orlistat works by decreasing the body's absorption of fat in the gastrointestinal tract. It frequently has the additional benefit of lowering cholesterol. Unfortunately, these benefits come at a price: fat that isn't absorbed by your body has to be eliminated, and this elimination results in oily stools, an urgent need to move your bowels that can cause incontinence, intestinal gas with discharge, abdominal pain, and diarrhea. Many people quit taking orlistat because of these embarrassing side effects. Orlistat also decreases the absorption of fat-soluble vitamins, so you need to take a vitamin supplement. Recently the FDA reported that it is looking into reports of liver damage in people taking orlistat, but it has not yet recommended any changes in the drug's use.

## Diet Composition

Is there an optimum diet for women with PCOS? We know that women with PCOS need a diet that controls weight, decreases insulin resistance, and maintains healthy cholesterol levels. There are few studies out there that examine exactly what that diet should look like, but there is some expert agreement. Ideally, you want a diet composed of low-fat foods, vegetable proteins, and foods that have a low glycemic index.

We are all familiar with the concept of a low-fat diet for cardiovascular health and of the importance of avoiding saturated fats, especially trans fats (also known as partially hydrogenated oils). Trans fats not only raise low-density lipoprotein (LDL, "bad" cholesterol); they also lower high-density lipoprotein (HDL, "good"

# Transtheoretical Model of Change

This model may help you understand the stages you go through as you try to change your eating behaviors. It sounds like an intimidating phrase but it's an easy concept. It views change as a process driven by **your intention to do things differently** rather than by outside forces. The path through the six stages is not a straight line from here to there, people often move back and forth between the stages before reaching the final stage of termination. So don't get down on yourself if you slip back occasionally. Each time you slip you are better armed to move forward again; you've learned from previous attempts and have more insight and information for the next round. At times you'll feel discouraged, but remember that it's a process and that if you just keep moving, you will get there.

### Precontemplation
Doing just fine—no need to change, thank you very much. There are people in much worse shape than I am. I've tried in the past and nothing ever works anyway, so the heck with it.

### Contemplation
Hmmm…I am overweight; maybe I should do something about it. But I don't want to give up my favorite foods. But I would feel so much better. I can't exercise every day. Who has the time? Maybe in six months, when things settle down…

### Preparation
I will start a diet after next week. I'll ask my friend at work to walk at lunch every day. I tried that low-carbohydrate diet last year but it didn't last. I'll take a look at the low-fat diet.

### Action
I'm eating a low-fat diet and walking three miles every day. It's really hard, especially when everyone else goes out for cheeseburgers at lunchtime and I'm walking around the parking lot instead. But I'm doing it.

### Maintenance
Sometimes I would love a cheeseburger, but not as much as I used to. I know I can say no to food like that now. I just have to make sure I keep it up. I make walking a priority every day; it's gotten so that I hate to miss it, I feel so much better when I walk every day.

### Termination
I can't remember the last time I had a cheeseburger and fries. I don't even want them. The thought of all that fat and grease…yuck! I don't let anything get in the way of my morning walk.

## What Nurses Know...

When it comes to weight loss, it is how much you eat that matters. However, when it comes to factors such as insulin resistance and cholesterol levels, it is what you eat that matters.

cholesterol). Fried foods, baked goods, margarine, and shortening often contain trans fats. Check the labels of processed foods, as manufacturers are now required by law to list trans fats. Several cities—New York, Boston, and Philadelphia, to name just three—have banned the use of trans fats in restaurant food, and others are in the process of doing so. The proportion of trans fats in your daily diet should be less than 1 percent.

People on very-low-carbohydrate diets usually consume meat—often quite a large quantity of meat—as their primary protein source. They may be successful at losing weight, but their LDL level remains the same—worse, it might actually go up. A higher intake of meat has also been associated with other negative health effects, including cancers of the digestive system, kidney disease, heart disease, and osteoporosis (thin bones that can break easily). Vegetable proteins are better than animal proteins (meat): they have a positive effect on cholesterol levels and have been shown to lower blood pressure in people with high blood pressure. Recent evidence shows that a low-carbohydrate diet that is high in vegetable proteins is best for lowering cholesterol levels. Along with the benefit of less saturated fats and cholesterol, this type of diet has a much higher fiber content than one in which meat is the main source of protein.

Much attention is now being paid to the glycemic index of foods, and especially to its effect on insulin resistance and diabetes control. The glycemic index ranks foods on a scale from 1 to 100 according to how much they affect glucose and insulin levels in the blood. A food that raises blood glucose quickly has a high glycemic index. Foods that are converted to glucose slowly have a low glycemic index. Maintaining a low-glycemic-index diet lowers insulin levels and decreases insulin resistance. It has also been shown to lower LDL levels and blood pressure.

Foods higher in fat and protein generally have a lower glycemic index. Fiber content also lowers a food's glycemic index. Many people still think that so-called simple sugars have the worst effect on blood sugar levels, but we now know that isn't true. Some complex carbohydrates, including potatoes and white bread, have a higher glycemic index than some candy products. However, you need to pay attention to more than just the glycemic index when choosing foods. Even if a candy bar has a low glycemic index it still has a lot of calories and no nutritional value. Look for the glycemic index symbol, a circle with a large G in the middle, which indicates that the food has been tested and meets international standards as a low-glycemic-index food.

*I didn't know anything about the glycemic index before. Now I look for the GI symbol on packages when I shop and I always read food labels. A lot of times you're really surprised. Like Frosted Flakes is one of the lowest cereals! I haven't eaten them for years—I bought*

## What Nurses Know . . .

*About now you're probably thinking, Who can keep track of all of this? The answer is a nutritionist. Schedule a couple of visits with a nutritionist to help you develop the diet plan that is best for you.*

*Many health insurance companies will cover nutrition counseling when there is a related diagnosis, such as glucose intolerance or pre-diabetes. Talk to your provider about getting a referral.*

*two big boxes! I definitely feel better when I'm sticking to my diet; when I don't, I have no energy to do anything.   AMY*

*I feel best when I stick to low carbs—I needed to become almost a vegetarian. It was like carbs were my enemy.   STEPHANIE*

Each person is different. If you are currently following a diet that works for you stick with it. If you are struggling with weight control and other PCOS symptoms try making the following changes in your diet:

- Eat about 40 percent carbohydrates.
- Choose carbohydrates that have a low glycemic index and avoid those that have a high glycemic index.
- Restrict your intake of animal proteins and increase your intake of vegetable proteins.
- Increase fiber in your diet to 30 grams daily.
- Don't eat carbohydrates alone; combine them with a protein or fat.
- Eat regular, small meals.
- Drink eight 8-ounce cups of noncaffeinated fluid throughout the day.

## What Nurses Know...

*Always read food labels; there are some real surprises out there. The marketing of certain foods can lead to misunder-standings about their supposed health benefits. Along with calorie counts, compare fiber, sugar, carbohydrate, fat (all kinds), protein, and sodium content as well as vitamin and mineral values.* **Make sure you look at serving size:** *serving size varies, which makes a big difference in actual values.*

## Calculating Carbohydrate Intake

Use the following calculation to work out how many grams of carbohydrates you should eat in a day to maintain a diet of 40 percent carbohydrates:

- Multiply your daily calorie intake by 0.4 (40 percent of your daily intake).
- Divide by 4 (carbohydrates average four calories per gram).

You can also use this formula to calculate your daily allowance of fat and protein. Just substitute the decimal number that goes with the desired percentage of daily intake (0.2 for 20 percent, 0.3 for 30 percent, etc.) in the first step and in the second step divide by 9 for fat and 4 for protein.

## Exercise

Exercise has multiple benefits for women with PCOS. It helps with weight control. Studies have found that when people engage in regular moderate exercise they lose more weight than if they just reduce their calorie intake and that they will lose a modest amount of weight even without cutting back on calories. Exercise also reduces the body's natural tendency to restore lost weight. Exercise improves the health of your heart and lungs. And in women with PCOS exercise raises SHBG. (Remember from Chapter 1 that the higher your SHBG, the lower your testosterone.) Exercise also reduces insulin resistance. This effect on SHBG and insulin resistance is separate from the effect of weight loss.

The current recommendation for adults is 30 minutes of moderate-intensity exercise five to seven days a week. However, to lose weight and maintain that loss you will need to increase that to at least 60 minutes five days a week or 40 minutes seven days a week.

Sounds like a lot, doesn't it? It is doable. Start slowly and build up to an hour a day. It doesn't have to be a continuous hour of exercise, but studies show that you need to exercise for at least 10 minutes at a time for it to be helpful. You could walk for 15 minutes four times a day or take a half-hour run in the morning and a half-hour walk at lunchtime. Playing tennis, swimming,

• • • • • • • • • • • • • • • • • • • • • • • • • • • •

## How Intense Is Moderate Intensity?

How do you tell the intensity level of your exercise? One way is to check your heart rate. For moderate intensity aim for a heart rate that is 50 to 70 per cent of your maximum heart rate, using the following calculation:

- Subtract your age from 220 to get your maximum heart rate (in beats per minute).
- Multiply that number by 0.5 to get the lower limit and by 0.7 for the upper limit.
- The result is the range you want your heart rate to be in during moderate-intensity exercise.

**Example**
You're 20 years old.

- Subtract 20 from 220 for a maximum heart rate of 200 beats per minute.
- Multiply 200 by 0.5 for a lower limit of 100 and by 0.7 for an upper limit of 140.
- You should keep your heart rate between 100 and 140 beats per minute for moderate-intensity exercise.

A couple of other methods don't require all these calculations and trying to take your pulse while you are exercising:

- If you're a walker get a pedometer. One hundred steps a minute represents a moderate level of intensity, so aim for 1,500 steps in 15 minutes.
- If you can easily carry on a conversation during the activity, your exercise intensity level is low. If you can carry on a conversation but not easily, your exercise intensity is moderate. If you can't carry on a conversation because you're too out of breath to speak, your exercise intensity is vigorous (too high unless you're an athlete or exceptionally fit).

So aim for that talking-with-difficulty stride. Of course, you won't want to try this method if your exercise is swimming!

**Remember: If you haven't been exercising start off slowly and build up your intensity level and the duration over time.**

taking the stairs instead of the elevator, jogging the dog instead of walking the dog—there are many ways to get that hour in.

Start by turning off the television. Television watching is a marker of an inactive lifestyle. If you spend two hours a day watching television, you are 23 percent more likely to be obese and 14 percent more likely to have diabetes than someone who watches no television.

Exercise is also a great stress buster. It will help you deal with the frustrations of your day and the difficulties related to PCOS. Exercise gives you a real sense of control over your life. You are doing it; with each step you are getting closer to your goals.

**One final word: patience. Lifestyle changes require persistence. It will take time to reverse symptoms, and you may not see any real differences for months. But stick with it and improvement will come.**

## Resources

### American Dietetic Association
The public information section offers comprehensive information about nutrition, diet and weight control among other topics.
www.eatright.org/

### American Heart Association
The Healthy Lifestyle section has information and tools for healthy eating, managing your weight, and exercise and fitness as well as women and heart disease.
www.amhrt.org/

### Centers for Disease Control: Healthy Weight
Web site on weight control offering a broad range of information on reaching and maintaining a healthy weight.
www.cdc.gov/healthyweight/index.html

### FDA: Make Your Calories Count
An interactive site where you can learn how to plan a healthy diet and manage your calorie intake.
www.fda.gov/Food/LabelingNutrition/ConsumerInformation/ucm114022.htm

### Glycemic Index Foundation and the GI Symbol Program
Information on the glycemic index and a database of the glycemic index values of specific foods.
www.gisymbol.com.au/index.htm

### Nutrition.gov
A gateway site to access all the food and nutrition information the federal government has, including food ingredients and weight management.
www.nutrition.gov/

### Obesity Society
A scientific organization working to enhance understanding, prevention, and treatment of obesity. It has a "Consumer Information" section.
www.obesity.org/consumers/

### Shape Up America!
A nonprofit organization whose Web site has all kinds of information on healthy weight management, covering diet, exercise, and behavior.
www.shapeup.org/

### U.S. Department of Agriculture National Agricultural Library
Lists government Web sites dealing with nutrition, exercise, and food-related health information.
http://fnic.nal.usda.gov/nal_display/index.php?tax_level=1&info_center=4

### Weight Watchers
You do not have to be a member of Weight Watchers to access many of the features of their Web site including extensive information on weight management, helpful tips on things like food shopping and eating out, and healthy cooking ideas.
www.weightwatchers.com/index.aspx

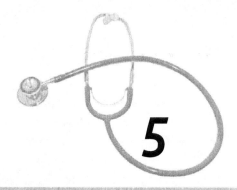

# 5

# Management of PCOS: Medications

*Things definitely improved after I started taking medications. My periods weren't so painful anymore and I had a lot more energy. And I didn't feel so depressed and ready to fly off the handle at any little thing. I still had good days and bad days, but the bad days weren't so bad like before.   AMY*

Medication strategy in PCOS is aimed at correcting the two factors believed to underlie the various symptoms of the disorder: high levels of androgens and insulin resistance. As discussed in Chapter 1, these two characteristics are tangled up in ways that are still not completely understood.

Two major classes of medications are used to manage PCOS: hormonal drugs and insulin-sensitizing drugs. These drugs are always prescribed in addition to the lifestyle changes discussed in the previous chapter, not in place of them. You will see the most improvement when you take control of your weight through lifestyle changes. The proper use of medications can build on this to get you closer to your goals.

Another class of medications, glucocorticoids (prednisone and dexamethasone), are used to treat high androgen levels related to problems with the adrenal glands, but they rarely have a place in the treatment of PCOS. They are not as effective as other medications for PCOS-related symptoms, and long-term use of glucocorticoids has serious harmful effects. If your provider prescribes them as part of your management plan you need to question the decision.

## What Nurses Know . . .

*General Medication Tips*

- *Always ask about generics; they're less expensive than brand-name drugs and almost always as effective.*
- *Keep an up-to-date record of all the medications you're on and show it to your provider whenever new medications are being prescribed or recommended, including over-the-counter medicines.*
- *Natural substances, herbal preparations, and supplements can interact with medications. Discuss any that you are taking with your provider and keep a list of them with your medication list.*
- *Always report any new or unusual symptoms to your provider.*
- *Allergic reactions can happen when you first take a medication or after you've been on it for some time. Stop your medication and call your provider if you have a rash, hives, or an unexplained cough. Call 911 if you experience unusual shortness of breath or wheezing, facial swelling, or swelling of the throat or tongue.*

## Hormonal Treatment

Hormonal treatment is the first-line medication for PCOS. It lowers androgen levels in one of two ways: some medications limit ovarian function to reduce the ovaries' production of testosterone; others interfere with the activity of testosterone. The two types of hormonal treatment medications are OCPs and antiandrogens. Usually these two types are taken together because each enhances the antiandrogen effects of the other so lower doses can be used and side effects are lessened.

### ORAL CONTRACEPTIVE PILLS

OCPs are effective at reducing hirsutism and acne, along with regulating periods. They suppress the levels of FSH and LH, which results in the ovaries secreting less testosterone. They raise the level of SHBG, so the level of free testosterone in the blood also drops. And there is the bonus, after four years of OCP use, of a much-lowered risk of endometrial and ovarian cancer—conditions that women with PCOS may be at higher risk for. Of course, OCPs are not an option if you're trying to get pregnant.

OCPs can have significant harmful effects, and they are not right for every woman. The most serious harmful effects are increased risks of blood clots, pancreatitis, and liver tumors. The overall risk of developing serious complications is low for most women—in fact, lower than with pregnancy. However, there are certain situations in which OCPs definitely should not be used.

If you have now or have in the past had any of the following conditions you should not use OCPs:

- A blood clotting disorder
- Cerebrovascular or coronary artery disease
- Uncontrolled hypertension
- Migraine headaches with aura or migraines that are persistent or severe
- Breast or uterine cancer
- Certain liver diseases or liver cancer
- Jaundice

You should also not be on OCPs if you are a smoker older than 35 years of age.

If you have now or have in the past had any of the following you need to discuss the risks with your provider and be extra careful about watching for side effects:

- Heart disease
- Kidney disease
- Gallbladder disease
- High blood pressure
- Hyperlipidemia
- Any migraine headaches
- Seizure disorders
- Asthma
- Obesity

You should not smoke if you are on OCPs. Smoking while on OCPs greatly increases your risk for developing a blood clot. Blood clots can cause a heart attack, a stroke, or a pulmonary embolism (when a clot travels to the lungs), any of which can be fatal. And it bears repeating that if you are older than 35 and smoke you should not be on OCPs, period.

There are many different OCPs out there, and choosing the right one is essential. The OCPs used to treat PCOS symptoms are combination pills: they contain both estrogen and progestin.

## What Nurses Know...

*OCPs are not interchangeable. They vary in the strength and types of estrogen and progestin formulas used. If you can't tolerate one OCP, try different formulas before giving up on using them altogether. For women with PCOS, pills that have nonandrogenic progestins may be preferred.*

Most progestins have some degree of androgenic effect, which limits their effectiveness in treating PCOS symptoms. Currently two progestins approved for use in the United States have no androgenic effects: norgestimate and desogestrel.

Drospirenone, a newer progestin approved by the FDA in 2001, actually has antiandrogenic effects. It is available as part of a combination OCP (Ocella, YAZ, or Yasmin). Many experts consider this the OCP of choice for most women with PCOS who are starting on OCP therapy. However, recently there have been reports of a greater risk of blood clots and strokes in women taking these pills than with other OCPs. Experts disagree about the accuracy of these reports, and two new studies have shown different results. If you are already doing well on your current treatment regimen stick with it. If you're not satisfied with your response to current treatment talk with your provider about the benefits of using an OCP containing drospirenone. Ask your provider for the latest information on the question of an increased risk.

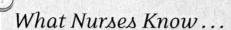

## What Nurses Know . . .

Be sure you tell providers if you are taking an OCP. OCPs should be included on your list of medications. They can interact with other medications, so providers need to know you are on them when prescribing. Also, certain medications may decrease the effectiveness of OCPs while you're taking them.

**You must use an alternate method of birth control while taking antibiotics and for seven days after finishing the course.** Continue taking your pills but use a barrier method, such as condoms, in addition.

St. John's wort, a herbal product, also decreases the effectiveness of OCPs and should not be taken while you are taking OCPs unless you use an additional method of birth control.

## What Nurses Know...

Many women experience nausea when they first start on OCPs. Ask your provider for a prescription for an antiemetic medication; take a dose about half an hour before taking your first pill, and continue to do so for the first week or so. Taking your pill at bedtime or with food will help also.

OCPs are usually started on the first day of the menstrual cycle. If your periods are irregular the pills can be started at any time, but you must first have a pregnancy test (no matter how unlikely you think it is that you are pregnant) and then use an alternate method of birth control for the first week. Take your pill at the same time every day, preferably at night (you'll sleep through any nausea or headaches).

A gap of 36 hours between taking two pills counts as a missed dose. (For example, if you take one pill at 9:00 A.M. on Wednesday and then your next pill at 10:00 P.M. on Thursday, you have missed a dose.) Any time you miss a dose, even one, you should use an alternate method of birth control for seven days. Missed doses only apply to the active pills in your pack; if you are using a 28-day prescription pack the last seven pills (a different color, usually white) are placebos, and missing any of those has no effect. Just be sure to stay on schedule and start your next pack at the right time.

OCPs can have uncomfortable side effects, including headaches, nausea, dizziness, breast tenderness, and breakthrough bleeding; these often subside after the first few months. The benefits of OCPs in women with PCOS make it worthwhile to try to see it through these initial discomforts. Of course, if the side effects are severe or interfere with your normal activities and quality of life, talk to your provider about trying a different formula or therapy. Occasionally women who wear contact lenses

## Missed Dose Schedule

- One pill missed: take the missed pill as soon as possible. If you remember it the next day, take two pills that day then resume your regular schedule.
- Two consecutive pills missed: take two pills a day for two days then resume your regular schedule. If you miss two consecutive pills during the third week of your prescription pack call your provider for directions.
- Three consecutive pills missed: call your provider for directions.

Always use an alternate birth control method for seven days after any missed dose.

experience eye discomfort; using a wetting solution more often usually takes care of this, so it is unlikely that you will have to choose between using contact lenses and taking OCPs.

Certain symptoms should never be ignored because they may signal one of the dangerous side effects of OCPs. If you have any of the following symptoms stop taking OCPs and contact your provider immediately. If your provider is not available go to an emergency room.

- Sudden numbness or weakness, especially on one side of the body only
- Chest pain or pressure
- Shortness of breath
- Coughing up blood
- New or unusually severe headache
- Severe abdominal pain
- Swelling in your feet or hands
- Redness, pain, or swelling in your lower leg
- Blurred vision, flashing lights, or blind spots

If you have any of the following symptoms continue taking your OCP but follow up with your provider right away:

- Abdominal pain
- Vaginal discharge

- A lump in your breast
- Two consecutive missed periods after a regular monthly pattern has been established

If you are on antiandrogens and stop OCPs you must start another reliable method of birth control right away.

You need to schedule a follow-up visit with your provider three months after starting OCPs and annually thereafter. Be sure to perform monthly breast self-exams while on OCPs. Remember that OCPs do not protect you from HIV or other sexually transmitted diseases, so use appropriate protection when having sex.

### ANTIANDROGENS

Antiandrogens are medications that block the action of testosterone. As discussed in Chapter 1, hormones don't have any activity of their own; their function is to regulate the activity of their target cells. They do this by attaching to receptors on the target cells. Antiandrogens work by competing with testosterone for these androgen receptors. When an antiandrogen molecule attaches to a receptor, no testosterone molecule can attach to the same receptor. If enough receptor sites are occupied by antiandrogens, then even if testosterone is present in the blood it cannot carry out its intended function.

**Spironolactone (Aldactone).**    Spironolactone is the preferred antiandrogen for the treatment of PCOS. It has been around for many years and has been shown to be safe and effective for treating the symptoms of PCOS. When spironolactone is taken with OCPs the effects of both are enhanced, so they are usually prescribed together. Spironolactone can cause frequent periods, and taking

• • • • • • • • • • • • • • • • • • • • • • • • • •

### Alert

You must use a reliable, effective method of birth control when taking antiandrogens. Antiandrogens can cause abnormal development of the genitalia in a male fetus.

ted death. Women with PCOS are at a higher

metabolic syndrome. (For further informa-

)

sitizing agent most commonly used in the

is metformin (Glucophage). Use in women

her group of insulin-sensitizing medications,

, has not been as well studied, and more

before they can be recommended as first-line

idinediones are also known to cause birth

used only in women who are not planning to

Use of metformin during pregnancy is consid-

ulin-sensitizing agent is part of your manage-

ost likely be metformin.


dication used in the treatment of diabetes that

duction of glucose by the liver and improves

sue cells to insulin. It interrupts the hyperin-

en feedback loop. Lower insulin levels in the

eased androgen levels. Decreased androgen

ight loss, improvement in symptoms such as

e, and increased fertility rates.

ot a magic pill. In fact, it is not as effective

e lifestyle changes discussed in the previous

s more often than not improve life for women

lly when used in combination with other treat-

are one of the majority of women with PCOS

intolerance (mildly elevated blood glucose lev-

ws that it may decrease your risk for diabetes

drome. It also has benefits if you are trying to

ussed in detail in Chapter 9).

dication, metformin has side effects, some

uite disruptive and unpleasant. Most women

degree of gastrointestinal distress when they

ormin, including bloating, nausea, vomiting,

OCPs has the added benefit of controlling this side effect. And because you should not get pregnant while you're taking antiandrogens, taking OCPs with spironolactone, or any antiandrogen, serves as a reliable method of birth control as well.

Spironolactone is a potassium-sparing diuretic: it gets rid of water but not potassium. Because elevated potassium levels can be harmful, you must avoid eating large quantities of foods that are high in potassium while taking spironolactone. Foods high in potassium include potatoes, citrus fruits, bananas, and tomatoes. You don't have to avoid them completely; just don't overdo it. Check the label of vitamin-enriched drinks and vitamin tablets for potassium as well.

Diuretics can cause low blood pressure and lightheadedness because your body is getting rid of more water than usual. If you experience lightheadedness after starting spironolactone drink extra fluid and get your blood pressure checked. Make sure you stay well hydrated in hot weather or when exercising. Always inform your provider about any changes in how you feel after starting a new treatment or medication.

**Cyproterone Acetate.** Cyproterone acetate is a progestin with antiandrogenic actions that is used in Europe and Canada to treat conditions associated with high androgen levels. It is available as a single drug and also as the progestin component in a

*What Nurses Know ...*

*Most salt substitutes contain potassium. Do not use them if you are taking spironolactone.*

*If you are restricting salt (sodium) in your diet try using other spices to season your food. Garlic, ground pepper, tarragon, oregano, nutmeg, and cinnamon are excellent choices to add flavor and zing to dishes.*

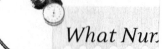

*What Nurses Know . . .*

*Take spironolactone early in the day so you're not getting up during the night to use the bathroom.*

combination OCP. The lower dose of cyproterone found in the OCP form makes it less effective than using the single drug form with a separate estrogen pill. In the United States cyproterone is approved only for treatment of severe hirsutism; however, some providers will prescribe it off-label to treat acne and mild to moderate hirsutism in women with PCOS. As with other antiandrogens, you should not get pregnant while on cyproterone.

**Finasteride.** Finasteride is not an antiandrogen, but it works to block the effects of androgens by interfering with the conversion of testosterone to dihydrotestosterone. Dihydrotestosterone is the hormone that binds with androgen receptors and stimulates many of the androgen-dependent actions in the body. Finasteride is not as effective as other antiandrogens for most symptoms of PCOS. It also has a greater potential for feminization of a male fetus than the others, so it is not considered a drug of choice. You should not take this medication if you are trying to conceive or are currently pregnant, and you must be on a reliable method of birth control if you do take it. It also should not be used if you are breastfeeding.

**Flutamide.** Flutamide is an antiandrogen that is very effective at reducing hirsutism. Unfortunately it has been known to cause severe and even fatal liver damage and so is rarely used. In the United States it is approved for use only in the treatment of prostate cancer. If your provider prescribes this drug off-label for hirsutism, ask why it is being chosen over other, less risky options.

---

cardiovascu
risk for dev
tion, see Cha

The insu
treatment o
with PCOS o
thiazolidine
research is n
treatment. T
defects, so th
become preg
ered safe. If a
ment plan, it

**METFORMIN**
Metformin is
suppresses th
the response
sulinemia-an
blood lead to
levels result i
hirsutism and

Metformin
a treatment a
chapter. But it
with PCOS, esp
ments. And if
who have gluco
els), research s
and metabolic
get pregnant (d

Like every
of which can b
experience som
start taking me

*What Nur*

**Off-Label Prescr**
*When the FDA a
turer to agree c
cific informatio
and administra
approved use of
have shown to b
Prescribing
approved use i
their profession
they decide to p
common and le
fessionals, pha
cies about the p
If your prov
decision should
think an off-la
gather informa
open a discuss*

Insulin-sensitizi
response of tissu
Insulin-sensitizi
benefits. They l
tance, which res
androgen levels
quences related
the presence of a
cate an increase

OCPs has the added benefit of controlling this side effect. And because you should not get pregnant while you're taking antiandrogens, taking OCPs with spironolactone, or any antiandrogen, serves as a reliable method of birth control as well.

Spironolactone is a potassium-sparing diuretic: it gets rid of water but not potassium. Because elevated potassium levels can be harmful, you must avoid eating large quantities of foods that are high in potassium while taking spironolactone. Foods high in potassium include potatoes, citrus fruits, bananas, and tomatoes. You don't have to avoid them completely; just don't overdo it. Check the label of vitamin-enriched drinks and vitamin tablets for potassium as well.

Diuretics can cause low blood pressure and lightheadedness because your body is getting rid of more water than usual. If you experience lightheadedness after starting spironolactone drink extra fluid and get your blood pressure checked. Make sure you stay well hydrated in hot weather or when exercising. Always inform your provider about any changes in how you feel after starting a new treatment or medication.

**Cyproterone Acetate.** Cyproterone acetate is a progestin with antiandrogenic actions that is used in Europe and Canada to treat conditions associated with high androgen levels. It is available as a single drug and also as the progestin component in a

## What Nurses Know...

Most salt substitutes contain potassium. Do not use them if you are taking spironolactone.

If you are restricting salt (sodium) in your diet try using other spices to season your food. Garlic, ground pepper, tarragon, oregano, nutmeg, and cinnamon are excellent choices to add flavor and zing to dishes.

*What Nurses Know . . .*

Take spironolactone early in the day so you're not getting up during the night to use the bathroom.

combination OCP. The lower dose of cyproterone found in the OCP form makes it less effective than using the single drug form with a separate estrogen pill. In the United States cyproterone is approved only for treatment of severe hirsutism; however, some providers will prescribe it off-label to treat acne and mild to moderate hirsutism in women with PCOS. As with other antiandrogens, you should not get pregnant while on cyproterone.

**Finasteride.** Finasteride is not an antiandrogen, but it works to block the effects of androgens by interfering with the conversion of testosterone to dihydrotestosterone. Dihydrotestosterone is the hormone that binds with androgen receptors and stimulates many of the androgen-dependent actions in the body. Finasteride is not as effective as other antiandrogens for most symptoms of PCOS. It also has a greater potential for feminization of a male fetus than the others, so it is not considered a drug of choice. You should not take this medication if you are trying to conceive or are currently pregnant, and you must be on a reliable method of birth control if you do take it. It also should not be used if you are breastfeeding.

**Flutamide.** Flutamide is an antiandrogen that is very effective at reducing hirsutism. Unfortunately it has been known to cause severe and even fatal liver damage and so is rarely used. In the United States it is approved for use only in the treatment of prostate cancer. If your provider prescribes this drug off-label for hirsutism, ask why it is being chosen over other, less risky options.

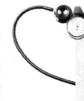

## What Nurses Know . . .

### Off-Label Prescribing

When the FDA approves a drug it works with the manufacturer to agree on the drug's labeling, which provides specific information about use, including indications, dosage, and administration. Labeling describes in detail the FDA-approved use of the drug and is based on what clinical trials have shown to be safe and effective.

Prescribing a drug for something other than an FDA-approved use is called off-label prescribing. Providers use their professional judgment, expertise, and experience when they decide to prescribe something off-label. This practice is common and legal, but there is debate among health care professionals, pharmaceutical companies, and regulatory agencies about the practice.

If your provider is going to prescribe a drug off-label, this decision should first be discussed in depth with you. If you think an off-label use of a drug may be beneficial to you, gather information about it to share with your provider and open a discussion.

## Insulin-Sensitizing Agents

Insulin-sensitizing agents are medications that improve the response of tissue cells to insulin. This lowers insulin resistance. Insulin-sensitizing agents have both short-term and long-term benefits. They lower androgen levels by lowering insulin resistance, which results in improvement in symptoms related to high androgen levels. They also decrease the risk of long-term consequences related to metabolic syndrome. Metabolic syndrome is the presence of a specific group of risk factors that together indicate an increased risk for diabetes, cardiovascular disease, and cardiovascular-related death. Women with PCOS are at a higher risk for developing metabolic syndrome. (For further information, see Chapter 7.)

The insulin-sensitizing agent most commonly used in the treatment of PCOS is metformin (Glucophage). Use in women with PCOS of another group of insulin-sensitizing medications, thiazolidinediones, has not been as well studied, and more research is needed before they can be recommended as first-line treatment. Thiazolidinediones are also known to cause birth defects, so they are used only in women who are not planning to become pregnant. Use of metformin during pregnancy is considered safe. If an insulin-sensitizing agent is part of your management plan, it will most likely be metformin.

### METFORMIN

Metformin is a medication used in the treatment of diabetes that suppresses the production of glucose by the liver and improves the response of tissue cells to insulin. It interrupts the hyperinsulinemia–androgen feedback loop. Lower insulin levels in the blood lead to decreased androgen levels. Decreased androgen levels result in weight loss, improvement in symptoms such as hirsutism and acne, and increased fertility rates.

Metformin is not a magic pill. In fact, it is not as effective a treatment as the lifestyle changes discussed in the previous chapter. But it does more often than not improve life for women with PCOS, especially when used in combination with other treatments. And if you are one of the majority of women with PCOS who have glucose intolerance (mildly elevated blood glucose levels), research shows that it may decrease your risk for diabetes and metabolic syndrome. It also has benefits if you are trying to get pregnant (discussed in detail in Chapter 9).

Like every medication, metformin has side effects, some of which can be quite disruptive and unpleasant. Most women experience some degree of gastrointestinal distress when they start taking metformin, including bloating, nausea, vomiting, flatulence (gas), and diarrhea. You can often lessen some of the initial side effects by starting at a lower dose and working your way up to the required dose, giving your body time to adjust to the medication.

> *When I first started metformin it was really rough. It seemed like I was in the bathroom every half hour for the first two to three weeks. Then my body got used to it and I was fine. If I miss a day though I'll have a problem when I take it the next day.   AMY*

> *It took me about a month or two to get used to taking the metformin. At first I was running to the bathroom constantly but after I started eating really good it started to get easier. Even now if I eat really, really bad I'm in the bathroom paying for it for a couple of days. In a way it's kind of a good thing because it actually helps me maintain the way I want to be eating.   STEPHANIE*

There is a small risk of a serious condition known as lactic acidosis developing in people who take metformin, especially those with kidney or liver disease. Make sure your provider checks your kidney and liver function before starting you on metformin and annually after that. And keep yourself well hydrated: you're more likely to develop lactic acidosis while on metformin if you are dehydrated.

## Alert

If you are on metformin report any of the following symptoms to your provider immediately:

- Unexplained muscle aches
- Malaise
- Unexplained rapid breathing
- Unusual sleepiness, difficulty staying awake or being awoken

These can be early symptoms of lactic acidosis.

## What Nurses Know . . .

### What to Ask When Medications Are Prescribed

- Should I take this with or without food?
- Should I take this at a certain time of day?
- What should I do if I miss a dose?
- Is it okay to drink alcohol while I'm on this medication?
- Will this medication affect my birth control pill's effectiveness?
- What are the most common side effects?
- Is there anything I can do to prevent the side effects?
- Are there any danger signs I need to watch for, and what do I do if they occur?
- Is there anything I need to avoid while on this medication (e.g., certain foods, sun exposure)?
- How long should I expect to be on this medication?
- Is it safe to get pregnant while on this medication?

## Resources

Be careful when looking up medication information on the Internet. Many sites are sponsored by drug companies and other sites, such as WebMD, have both reliable objective information and sponsored links. Information sponsored by drug companies is likely to be biased in favor of their drugs.

### Medline Plus

A service of the National Institutes of Health, this site offers information on a comprehensive list of medications.
http://www.nlm.nih.gov/medlineplus/druginformation.html

### FDA: Information for Consumers

This FDA site offers general information on medication use for consumers.
http://www.fda.gov/Drugs/ResourcesForYou/Consumers/default.htm

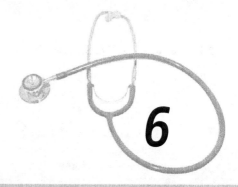

6

# Dealing With Body Image Issues

*You go to the doctor's office and in the waiting room are all these glamour magazines. Sometimes I want to run and hide and just not have to deal with it.   STEPHANIE*

Everywhere you turn you see her—posing on magazine covers, peering down from billboards, smiling from your television set— the ideal woman, thin and smooth skinned. It's hard enough for any woman to live up to the image, let alone someone dealing with PCOS-related body issues.

## Hirsutism

In our society the feminine ideal is hairless skin. Women get waxed, shaved, plucked, and lasered all over their bodies. They spend time and money to remove every trace of stray hair outside

● ● ● ● ● ● ● ● ● ● ● ● ● ● ● ● ● ● ● ● ● ● ● ● ● ● ● ● ●

## Stat Facts

- There are about 50 million hair follicles covering the body.
- Of these, 20 percent are on your scalp. There are none on your palms, the soles of your feet, or your lips.
- Most of our hair follicles are present at birth, and we begin to lose follicles after age 40.
- The growth cycles of individual hair follicles differ; it appears that hair grows continuously, but only some follicles are in the growth phase at any given time.

those on their head. No wonder hirsutism is reported as the most distressing symptom of PCOS.

Women with hirsutism often refer to themselves as "freaks" and invest considerable time, energy, and money trying to look "normal." They may go to great lengths to hide the truth about their bodies, avoiding situations where their secret could be revealed and concealing their daily hair removal rituals from everyone, even partners, fearful that others may discover they're not "real women."

*I started noticing the extra hair growth when I was a teenager. I'm very self-conscious about it. I never wear a bathing suit at the beach; I always wear shorts. Even if I shave that morning it doesn't help.*　AMY

### BACKGROUND

Hirsutism is defined as the excessive growth of terminal hair in a male distribution pattern in women. There are two types of hair on the body: vellus and terminal. Vellus hair is soft, fine, short, colorless hair on areas of the body we think of as hairless. Terminal hair is coarse, long, and pigmented. Scalp hair, eyebrows, and eyelashes are examples of terminal hair. At puberty increased androgen levels in both girls and boys result in the growth of terminal hair in the pubic region and axilla, where hair

### Stat Fact

● Hirsutism affects about 8 percent of women in the United States (more than four million women).

follicles are very sensitive to androgens. Other areas, those associated with male-pattern hair growth, such as the face and chest, are not as sensitive to androgens and require much higher levels for terminal hair growth.

Although the growth of sexual hair is dependent on androgens, the degree of hirsutism is not related to the degree of androgen excess. The majority of hirsutism is associated with high androgen levels, but it can also present in women with normal androgen levels (idiopathic hirsutism). On the other hand, some women with high levels of androgens have no hirsutism at all. This suggests that other factors may contribute to the development of hirsutism. It is known that increased sensitivity of the hair follicle to androgens is one factor, and research suggests that a high level of insulin in the blood is another.

The degree of hirsutism is measured using the Ferriman-Gallwey scale. A pictorial scale is used to assign a rating from 0 (no abnormal hair growth) to 4 (extensive abnormal hair growth)

## What Nurses Know...

*The Ferriman-Gallwey scale is a subjective tool. Each provider uses his or her own judgment when assigning a score. One provider's 2 may be another's 3. Make sure everyone involved in your care is working from a common copy of your scorecard; otherwise it is difficult to measure progress, and treatment decisions may be based on inaccurate information.*

for nine different areas of the body where excess hair growth occurs: above the lip and on the chin, chest, upper and lower abdomen, arms, groin/upper thigh, back, and buttocks. An overall score of 8 or more indicates hirsutism (though some providers use 6 as the cutoff).

### MANAGEMENT

The management of hirsutism varies according to the severity of each case. Mild hirsutism can often be treated with mechanical measures such as bleaching, shaving, electrolysis, and laser treatment. Moderate to severe hirsutism requires both systemic and mechanical approaches. Systemic measures include OCPs and antiandrogens. These stop the progression of terminal hair growth but do not reduce existing levels, so they should be combined with cosmetic measures.

There is one more effective management approach: weight loss. As mentioned in Chapter 4, weight loss lowers androgen levels and decreases hirsutism.

Keep in mind that it will take time for any systemic approach to have an effect. Hair goes through three phases: an active growth phase, a dormant phase, and finally a shedding phase. Any hair already present has to go through all three phases before you see a marked change. You can use mechanical measures to manage hirsutism until systemic treatments kick in.

## What Nurses Know . . .

*It's all about perception. No matter where you fall on the Ferriman-Gallwey scale, or any other measurement tool, the final judgment of severity lies with you. If you feel you have hair in places it doesn't belong and it's affecting your quality of life, then it's severe enough to be treated.*

## MECHANICAL HAIR REMOVAL

|  | Pros | Cons |
|---|---|---|
| Depilatories | Inexpensive<br>Do-it- yourself | Can cause chronic skin irritation<br>Overuse can result in worsening<br>of hair growth<br>Temporary |
| Shaving | Inexpensive<br>Do-it-yourself | Time-consuming<br>Temporary |
| Bleaching | Inexpensive<br>Do-it-yourself<br>No side effects when<br>used appropriately | Can be used only for very mild<br>local hair growth<br>Temporary |
| Plucking and<br>waxing | Inexpensive<br>Do-it-yourself | Can cause ingrown hairs<br>Can cause folliculitis (infection<br>of hair follicles)<br>Painful<br>Temporary |
| Electrolysis | Permanent | Painful<br>Expensive<br>Time-consuming<br>Only useful for small areas<br>Can cause skin irritation, burns,<br>and scarring |
| Laser<br>treatment | Permanent<br>Can treat large areas<br>of growth<br>Results in up to 30<br>percent reduction in<br>hair density | Painful<br>Expensive<br>Time-consuming<br>Can cause skin irritation, burns,<br>scarring, and loss of skin<br>pigmentation |

**Electrolysis.** Electrolysis destroys hair follicles by using a fine, sterile probe to deliver electricity into the hair follicle. It is very effective for small areas such as the chin and upper lip, but it has some drawbacks. It is painful: women describe the pain as feeling like a bee sting. It is time consuming: treatments for facial hair can take anywhere from 15 minutes to an hour each time. The number of treatments varies greatly among individuals, but it can take months or even a year or more to get adequate results, and periodic touch-ups are required after that. It is expensive, costing from $50 to $125 an hour depending on where you live.

There are also potential risks: electrolysis can cause local reactions, burns, and scarring. **Be sure you find a well-qualified technician.**

**Laser Treatment.**   For larger areas laser treatments are a better choice than electrolysis. Lasers use pulses of light to create heat that destroys the hair follicles. Light-skinned women with dark hair do best with laser treatments; they can be successfully treated using lower-energy light pulses. This doesn't mean laser treatment won't work for you if you have dark skin; just make sure the treatment uses lasers with built-in cooling devices to avoid skin damage, because you will need a higher temperature for a longer duration. Lasers can permanently reduce hair by about 30 percent within three or four treatments. But laser treatment, like electrolysis, is painful: the laser feels like a prolonged sharp sting. It is also expensive: depending on how extensive the treatment is, each session can cost hundreds of dollars.

Risks are similar to those with electrolysis, but laser treatment can also cause changes in the pigmentation of your skin. To prevent this you should avoid exposing the treated areas to sunlight for the duration of your treatments.

## What Nurses Know . . .

**Do not go bargain shopping for these procedures.** Make sure your technician has the proper credentials, training, and experience. Laser treatment is regulated in all states by the state medical board. Electrolysis is regulated in most states, and licenses are issued by the Barbering and Cosmetology or Health Department.

## TOPICAL PRESCRIPTION MEDICATIONS

Vaniqa is a prescription cream used to treat unwanted facial hair. It does not remove the hair, but it slows the growth and decreases the length of hair already present. It has some effect in about 60 percent of women, and about half of those show a marked improvement. You'll see the maximum improvement in anywhere from 8 to 24 weeks. The change is not permanent; once you stop using the cream, hair growth returns to its preuse rate. If you don't notice any improvement after four months of use, Vaniqa is not going to work for you.

Side effects reported with Vaniqa are most commonly related to skin irritation, such as burning and stinging. Use should be limited to the face because it is not known whether the increased absorption that would result from use over large areas of the body could be harmful.

*My OB/GYN told me to get electrolysis, that I'd be so happy with the results. I can't afford that! My insurance doesn't cover it. So, I just shave every day.   AMY*

## METFORMIN

Research has reported mixed results regarding the effectiveness of metformin for treatment of hirsutism. As high levels of insulin in the blood have been linked to the development of excess terminal hair it is logical to think that lowering insulin levels would be beneficial, and some studies bear this out. But a number of other studies have found no benefit. Until there is stronger evidence either way it is reasonable to use metformin (if tolerated well) as an additional therapy when OCPs and antiandrogens don't

● ● ● ● ● ● ● ● ● ● ● ● ● ● ● ● ● ● ● ● ● ● ● ● ● ●

## Money Matters

Health insurance does not cover cosmetic treatments. So even though hirsutism is a symptom of the medical condition of PCOS, treatment costs are not covered by most health insurance policies.

• • • • • • • • • • • • • • • • • • • • • • • • • • • •

## Alert

**Medications That Can Cause or Worsen Hirsutism**
- Anabolic steroids
- Reglan (metoclopramide, used to treat heartburn caused by gastric reflux)
- Aldomet (methyldopa, used to treat high blood pressure)
- Phenothiazines (organic compounds found in various antipsychotic and antihistaminic drugs)
- Progestins
- Serpasil (reserpine, used to treat hypertension)
- Testosterone

yield good results or when you aren't able to tolerate their side effects.

## Alopecia (Baldness)

Some women with PCOS have to deal with the other end of the spectrum as well: hair loss. The frustration of having too much hair where you don't want it is compounded by that of having too little hair where you do. Alopecia in women is typically characterized by a general thinning of hair over the entire scalp rather than the receding hairline seen in men.

Elevated levels of testosterone are usually the cause of alopecia in women with PCOS. Free testosterone in the blood is converted into dihydrotestosterone, which is the hormone that stimulates hair follicles to grow. Too much testosterone in a woman usually means too much hair growth—except on the scalp. In some people scalp hair follicles are oversensitive to testosterone, and higher levels cause the hair to fall out rather than grow. The reasons for this are not completely understood (beginning to sound familiar?), but it appears that there is a genetic predisposition toward baldness in both men and women. Usually in women it doesn't manifest because testosterone levels are low.

Some medications can also cause hair loss and baldness, among them isotretinoin, which is used to treat severe acne.

Acne is a common problem for women with PCOS, and a few may experience acne severe enough to require isotretinoin. If you notice hair loss after starting isotretinoin, the drug may be the culprit. If isotretinoin is recommended for you ask your provider about hair loss when discussing potential side effects. Hair loss is actually one of the less common side effects of isotretinoin, and usually (but not always) hair will grow back a few months after stopping the medication. (Use of isotretinoin is covered in detail in the section on acne below.)

As with hirsutism and other symptoms of PCOS, the first-line treatment for alopecia in women with PCOS is to lower androgen levels. This means lifestyle measures to start with, especially weight loss, and then medications such as OCPs, antiandrogens, and possibly metformin. If these measures don't yield satisfactory results, other treatment options are available. Currently only two medications are approved by the FDA for treatment of hair loss: minoxidil and finasteride. Of the two, only minoxidil is approved for use in women with alopecia.

**Minoxidil.** Minoxidil is a topical drug used to treat alopecia in men and women. It comes in either a foam or a solution and is applied directly to the scalp, usually twice a day. It takes a few months to see new hair growth, but hair loss should stop after the first two weeks. Minoxidil is effective only while you are using it; hair loss will resume a couple of months after stopping treatment. You can use minoxidil if you color, relax, or perm your hair, but you should wash your scalp well before applying hair products and should not use minoxidil for 24 hours before and after. Minoxidil can stain clothing and bed linens, so plan your applications so that your scalp is dry before dressing or going to bed. It takes four hours or so to dry, which may create some scheduling inconveniences.

Make sure you use minoxidil as directed and wash your hands well after each application. Minoxidil was originally developed as a powerful oral antihypertensive, and you may experience serious problems if too much is absorbed into your body,

## What Nurses Know...

*Always use topical medications as directed. When medication is applied to the skin some of it is absorbed into the body. If the medication is applied over a larger area of the body than it is intended for or more frequently than recommended, more will be absorbed into the body, increasing the risk of adverse side effects.*

especially if you have hypertension or heart disease. Minoxidil should not be used if you are trying to conceive or are pregnant or breastfeeding.

**Finasteride.** Finasteride is an antiandrogen that has been used with some success in men with alopecia. It is not approved by the FDA for use in women, but it is sometimes prescribed off-label for alopecia in women with PCOS. However, remember from Chapter 5 that finasteride can cause feminine characteristics in a male fetus; it should never be used if you are trying to conceive or are pregnant or breastfeeding.

### HAIR CARE AND PRODUCTS

A great many products out there are touted as treatments for hair loss, but there is no evidence to support these claims. Do not be taken in by advertisements. A number of over-the-counter hair products can make your hair *appear* thicker and fuller, but other than minoxidil and finasteride, no products are available that actually increase hair growth or stop hair loss.

Your hair care routine will not affect the rate of hair loss or hair growth, but it can make a big difference in the appearance of your existing hair, making it look thicker or thinner. Certain hair care routines, such as frequent blow-drying, bleaching, tight braiding, hot curlers, or flat plates, can cause dryness and

## Hair-Loss Myths

The following false claims are among those you will see used to promote products:

- Increasing blood flow to the scalp will stop hair loss and increase hair growth.
- You can increase the number of hair follicles on your scalp and thereby increase hair growth.
- Special hair products do not damage your hair and cause hair loss in the way that others do.
- Certain herbal products, vitamins, or natural supplements will stop hair loss or promote hair growth.
- Unplugging hair follicles will promote hair growth.

Again, there are products that will make your hair appear healthier and thicker, but they will not stop hair loss or promote hair growth.

damage the hair shaft, resulting in weak, brittle hair and thinner hair coverage. Some experts recommend that women with alopecia should wash their hair with a gentle shampoo every day. Hair looks fuller if it isn't weighed down by the buildup of dirt and oils. Other hair products make hair look thicker by roughening the hair cuticle. Hair color and perms also have this effect, but be careful not to overuse them and end up with damaged hair.

## Acne

It is normal for women to have some acne on and off from puberty to menopause. However, persistent, severe, or cystic acne is usually associated with high androgen levels. Hormonal treatment to lower androgen levels, such as OCPs and antiandrogens, is the foundation of treatment. Topical agents and systemic antibiotics are often used to supplement systemic treatment or as single therapy in pregnant women.

Acne originates in the sebaceous glands of the skin, most commonly on the face, chest, and back. Sebaceous glands are small oil-secreting glands that are usually attached to a hair follicle. They are present all over the skin, except on the palms of the

● ● ● ● ● ● ● ● ● ● ● ● ● ● ● ● ● ● ● ● ● ● ● ● ● ● ●

## Stat Facts

- Between 24 and 39 percent of women with PCOS have problems with acne.
- Between 70 and 87 percent of adolescents experience acne, with a peak incidence between 15 and 18 years of age.

hands and the soles of the feet, and are abundant on the face and scalp. Sebaceous glands secrete sebum, an oily, fatty substance that protects the skin by keeping it lubricated and preventing the loss of too much water. Testosterone causes sebaceous glands to enlarge and increases the production of sebum, which solidifies and clogs the hair follicle.

Clogged follicles form three different types of lesions: open or closed comedones or pimples. Comedones form when the glands are plugged with dried, discolored sebum, and they may be open (whiteheads) or closed (blackheads). The bacterium *Propionibacterium acnes*, which is present on the skin after puberty, multiplies in the presence of comedones and interacts with the sebum in them to cause an inflammatory response that forms pimples. Cystic acne is the severest form, characterized by the presence of deep, pus-filled, nodular pimples. It is important to treat moderate and severe acne to prevent permanent scarring.

● ● ● ● ● ● ● ● ● ● ● ● ● ● ● ● ● ● ● ● ● ● ● ● ● ●

## Myths About Acne

- Chocolate and greasy food cause acne.

There is no evidence that a particular food causes or worsens acne.

- Dirty skin causes acne.

Acne is not caused by dirty skin.

- Stress causes acne.

Stress does not cause acne, but it can have an effect on its severity.

## MANAGEMENT

Acne can be treated through two mechanisms: lowering androgen levels or inhibiting the inflammatory response. Usually a combination of these approaches is used, at least initially. Systemic agents such as hormonal medications and oral antibiotics are prescribed, along with topical agents such as retinoids and antibiotic creams.

> *I had really bad acne in high school but once I started the birth control pills and metformin and Aldactone it cleared up; plus they had me taking an acne medicine for about six months. It's been fine since.* AMY

### Systemic Treatment

*Hormonal Treatment.* OCPs and antiandrogens are the mainstay of treatment for acne in nonpregnant women. Both are very effective in decreasing acne. (Detailed information about these medications can be found in Chapter 5.)

*Oral Antibiotics.* Moderate to severe cases of acne usually require an oral antibiotic as part of the initial treatment. Oral antibiotics reduce the number of bacteria on the skin and calm the inflammatory response. Oral antibiotics are prescribed for about four to six months, and you should see improvement after four to six weeks. If there is no improvement after six months, the bacterium is probably resistant to the antibiotic and a different one will need to be tried. Treatment with oral antibiotics should be limited to six months to avoid the development of antibiotic resistance.

## Hormonal Medications Used in the Treatment of Acne

- Combination OCPs
- Spironolactone
- Cyproterone acetate

# Oral Antibiotics Used in the Treatment of Acne

### Tetracycline
- Most commonly prescribed oral antibiotic
- Should be taken on an empty stomach
- Can cause gastrointestinal upset
- Should not be taken after the expiration date; can become toxic
- Avoid sun exposure and use high sun protection factor (SPF) sunscreen when outside
- Usually will decrease acne by 50 percent after six weeks of treatment
- Not safe to use if you are pregnant
- Usually taken four times a day to start with and then once or twice a day for long-term treatment
- If you are taking OCPs for birth control, use an alternate method of contraception during the therapy and for one week after stopping medication

### Doxycycline and Minocycline
- Newer forms of tetracycline
- Can be taken with meals, which may help prevent gastrointestinal upset
- More expensive than tetracycline
- Need to be taken only once or twice a day
- Avoid sun exposure and use high SPF sunscreen when outside
- Can cause blue-gray discoloration of skin and teeth; taking ascorbic acid helps decrease tooth discoloration
- Rare instances of these drugs causing liver disease and autoimmune diseases, so your provider may get blood work to check your liver function or for any evidence of autoimmune diseases
- Should not be taken after the expiration date; can become toxic
- Not safe to use if you are pregnant
- If you are taking OCPs for birth control, use an alternate method of contraception during the therapy and for one week after stopping medication
- Minocycline is more effective and works faster and for longer than tetracycline or doxycycline
- Minocycline can have significant side effects, including severe reactions, dizziness, and lung and kidney problems

### Erythromycin
- More resistance than other choices
- Inexpensive
- Causes gastrointestinal side effects in most users
- Should be taken with food to reduce gastrointestinal upset
- Safe in pregnancy, so may be the only option if you are pregnant or attempting to conceive

### Clindamycin
- Oral form rarely used
- Long-term use can cause a serious form of colitis

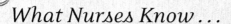

## What Nurses Know...

*Some medications must be taken on an empty stomach because the presence of food or certain liquids (such as dairy products) in the stomach will decrease their absorption and hence their effectiveness.*

### Tips for Taking Medications on an Empty Stomach

*Medications that need to be taken on an empty stomach should be taken one hour before or two hours after eating. Take the medication with a full glass of water.*

*Take the medication at least an hour before bedtime. Gravity aids digestion, and when you are lying down the medication can sit in your stomach longer or regurgitate into your esophagus and cause gastritis or esophagitis.*

*If you experience intolerable gastrointestinal side effects ask your provider whether there is a different medication you can use that does not cause gastrointestinal upset.*

*If all else fails you may have to take the medicine with a small amount of food rather than stop taking it altogether.*

Tetracycline is the most commonly prescribed oral antibiotic. Though resistance has developed, it is still a good first choice because it is generally effective and it's inexpensive.

*Isotretinoin.* Isotretinoin (Accutane) is a systemic retinoid that is very effective in the treatment of severe acne that does not respond to oral antibiotics. It works on all the factors that cause acne: it decreases the size of sebaceous glands, reduces sebum production, and lowers the number of bacteria on the skin.

However, isotretinoin is known to have a number of serious side effects. It causes significant birth defects if taken during pregnancy. In fact, the risk is so great that the FDA requires you and your provider to register in an electronic database before you can get a prescription for isotretinoin filled. Your provider and the pharmacist must confirm that you have had two negative pregnancy tests and are using two methods of birth control before dispensing the medication. The other major side effect is an increased rate of depression, psychosis, and suicide while taking the medication. Isotretinoin can also cause liver disease, visual problems, and eye ulcerations.

This doesn't mean that isotretinoin should not be used, but its use should be limited to severe cases of acne—and only after you have tried all the other options first. If you do decide to take isotretinoin, careful monitoring is required, including periodic blood tests. And remember: isotretinoin does not treat the underlying cause of acne in women with PCOS, while OCPs and antiandrogens do.

**Topical Agents.** Topical agents are medications that are applied directly to the skin. Like oral antibiotics they work by lowering bacteria levels and decreasing inflammation. Topical agents have the advantage over systemic treatments that they do not carry the risk of serious or unpleasant side effects, other than local reactions.

Among the most commonly used topical agents is benzoyl peroxide, a bactericide that is effective against a broad range of bacteria, including *Propionibacterium acnes.* It is the active ingredient in numerous over-the-counter products, including soaps, cleansers, liquids, lotions, creams, and masks. Benzoyl peroxide is relatively inexpensive. It is available in strengths from 2.5 to 20 percent, but using anything stronger than 5 percent is usually unnecessary. Stronger formulations rarely improve effectiveness, and they increase your risk of experiencing benzoyl peroxide's most common side effect: skin irritation. Benzoyl peroxide is not meant to be used as a spot treatment; you should apply it over the entire affected area. Be aware that it can bleach hair, clothes, and bed linens, so plan applications so that it will be completely dry before you get dressed or go to bed.

If your acne is moderate to severe benzoyl peroxide alone will not provide sufficient results. Benzoyl peroxide combined with topical antibiotics or retinoids is the most effective topical treatment for moderate to severe acne. Erythromycin and clindamycin are the most commonly used topical antibiotics. Treatment needs to continue for at least six to eight weeks.

Topical retinoids are a derivative of vitamin A. They improve acne through two actions: they decrease inflammation by increasing the turnover of skin cells, and they prevent the clogging of pores by decreasing sebum secretion. In combination treatments, these actions enhance the effectiveness of topical antibiotics by allowing them to penetrate deeper into skin pores. If you are using a topical retinoid alone ask your provider about prescribing a two-week course of antibiotics to prevent the flare-up of pimples that often accompanies retinoid therapy. Other side effects are skin irritation, sun sensitivity, and skin peeling. Topical retinoids can reduce acne by 40 to 70 percent. Of the available retinoids—tazarotene, tretinoin, and adapalene—tazarotene has been shown to be the most effective, but it also tends to cause more irritation than the others.

Topical antibiotics should always be used in combination with benzoyl peroxide, retinoids, or azelaic acid to increase their effectiveness and help prevent resistance. Azelaic acid is another antibacterial and anti-inflammatory agent. It is usually well tolerated, but women with dark complexions have to be careful in using it because it can cause hypopigmentation.

## Acanthosis Nigricans

Acanthosis nigricans is a brown or black velvety discoloration of the skin. It is usually seen in skin folds, especially around the neck and axilla, but it may appear on the thighs or genital area as well. It normally develops slowly and is associated with insulin resistance and diabetes. It is not harmful in and of itself. The strategies used to decrease insulin resistance—weight loss, diet, and medication—are effective for preventing and treating acanthosis nigricans, but if these measures fail then cosmetic procedures such as dermabrasion and laser therapy or medications used to treat acne can be helpful. Topical retinoids or over-the-counter creams containing salicylic acid or alpha hydroxy acids may lighten the areas. Severe acanthosis nigricans that doesn't respond to other treatments may respond to isotretinoin.

## Resources

### American Academy of Dermatology
The "Public Center" is a resource for reliable information on skin care in general, with links to information on acne. The site can also help you locate a reputable dermatologist in your area.
www.aad.org/public/index.html

### American Hair Loss Association
An organization that works to improve the lives of people affected by hair loss. The Webs ite has extensive information about hair loss, including a section specifically for women.
www.americanhairloss.org/

### MedlinePlus: Acne
A National Institutes of Health Web site on acne with numerous links to further information.
www.nlm.nih.gov/medlineplus/acne.html

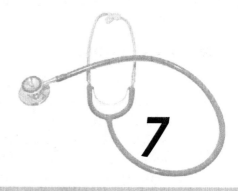

# The Big Three: Diabetes, Cardiovascular Disease, and Cancer

*The endocrinologist I'm seeing now got right down to the bottom line. She was honest with me. She said, "This is for the rest of your life. You don't want to die of a heart attack or cancer. You have to take care of yourself."* STEPHANIE

For a long time PCOS was thought to be a disorder only of the reproductive system, and management was focused on regulation of the menstrual cycle and helping women conceive. We now know that PCOS has serious implications for a woman's long-term health. The high insulin levels in the blood and insulin resistance associated with PCOS can put a woman at risk for metabolic syndrome and related cardiovascular disease. Women with PCOS are also known to have an increased risk of endometrial cancer.

Screening and preventive measures are important parts of your management plan. You and your provider must pay attention early and often to the metabolic symptoms of the disorder and to risk factors for the development of endometrial cancer. This is your best strategy for living a full, healthy life.

Almost 30 years before Stein and Leventhal published their report on the syndrome that came to be known as PCOS, a condition of excess androgens combined with diabetes in women had already been noted. This early association with diabetes was forgotten after Stein and Leventhal's report, and it wasn't until the 1980s, when the association between PCOS and insulin resistance was noted, that diabetes entered the PCOS picture again. Now we know that women with PCOS are at high risk for metabolic syndrome and its attendant health risks, particularly diabetes and cardiovascular disease.

It is important to note here that even though many factors place women with PCOS at higher risk for cardiovascular disease, the evidence about their actual risk of experiencing cardiovascular problems or dying as a result of a cardiovascular event such as a heart attack is not definitive. The risk appears to be slightly elevated, but not by as much as the number of risk factors present might lead one to expect. This is reassuring, but it does not mean you should be any less concerned about your cardiovascular health or lax in your prevention efforts. Experts agree that it is too soon to draw any conclusions and that more research is needed before we can know the full effect that PCOS will have on a woman's health and life 20, 30, or 40 years down the road. In the meantime, preventive measures are paramount in assuring the healthy, full life you desire.

• • • • • • • • • • • • • • • • • • • • • • • • • •

## Stat Facts

- Metabolic syndrome is present in about 40 percent of women with PCOS, almost twice the rate found in the general population.
- Diabetes mellitus type II is present in about 15 percent of women with PCOS, compared with 6 percent of the general population.

## Characteristics of Metabolic Syndrome

Metabolic syndrome is characterized by the presence of three or more of the following:

- Waist circumference 35 inches or more
- Fasting blood glucose 150 mg/dL or higher
- HDL cholesterol less than 50 mg/dL
- Blood pressure 130/85 mm Hg or higher

## Metabolic Syndrome

Metabolic syndrome is a combination of characteristics that put a person at higher risk for diabetes, cardiovascular disease, and cardiovascular mortality.

Let's look more closely at the characteristics of metabolic syndrome and how they relate to women with PCOS.

*Waist Circumference 35 Inches or More.* Central obesity is common in women with PCOS. People with central obesity carry their excess fat in the abdominal area, much of it surrounding the internal organs. Someone with central obesity has a higher risk of developing cardiovascular problems than an obese person whose excess fat is distributed throughout the body under the skin.

*Fasting Blood Glucose 150 mg/dL or Higher.* A fasting blood glucose concentration of 150 mg/dL is an indicator of diabetes. Women with PCOS are at high risk for developing diabetes. Simply put, over time the stressed pancreas is no longer able to compensate for the insulin resistance associated with PCOS by secreting more insulin, leading to impaired glucose tolerance. Without serious lifestyle changes, this impaired glucose tolerance will eventually lead to diabetes. It is estimated that 30 to 40 percent of women with PCOS have blood test results that indicate either impaired glucose tolerance or diabetes at the time of their diagnosis.

*HDL Cholesterol Less Than 50 mg/dL.* PCOS is associated with low HDL levels. HDL is known as "good cholesterol" because it helps mop up excess cholesterol along blood vessel walls and carry it back to the liver, where the digestive system takes over and gets rid of it. This helps prevent atherosclerosis, or the thickening of artery walls. HDL also helps ward off blood vessel constriction and injury. Thus, the higher your HDL level, the lower your risk of cardiovascular disease, including heart attack and stroke. Women with PCOS who have high levels of insulin in their blood, regardless of weight, tend to have lower HDL levels then those with normal levels of insulin. They also tend to have higher levels of LDL, or "bad cholesterol." The combination of high LDL levels and low HDL levels multiplies the risks associated with having either of them alone. Studies have determined that the high-risk lipid levels in women with PCOS are not explained by differences in body weight. These lipid abnormalities are found in both obese and lean women with PCOS. However, studies have reported that women with PCOS who are obese have worse levels than those who are not. In other words, lipid abnormalities are inherent in PCOS, and although obesity is not the cause of abnormal lipid levels in women with PCOS, it does have an important impact.

*Blood Pressure 130/85 mm Hg or Higher.* There are conflicting data about the association between PCOS and high blood pressure. Some studies have reported a higher rate of hypertension in women with PCOS regardless of age, weight, and glucose levels, but others have reported different results. Either way, studies have consistently shown that as women with PCOS age they are more likely to develop high blood pressure than women without PCOS who have an otherwise similar health profile.

It becomes clear now why women with PCOS have a higher risk of developing metabolic syndrome: all the characteristics associated with metabolic syndrome are commonly present in women with PCOS. In addition, there are other factors, independent of metabolic syndrome, that increase the risk of cardiovascular disease in women with PCOS: they may have decreased elasticity and increased inflammatory changes in their blood vessels, increased coronary artery calcification, and thickening of the inner lining of the carotid artery.

The good news is that despite the real increased risk of developing diabetes and cardiovascular disease associated with PCOS, there are actions you can take to lower your personal risk. It is within your control.

## MANAGING YOUR RISK PROFILE

**Lifestyle Changes.**  Weight control, good dietary patterns, and exercise are the cornerstones of risk prevention. The importance of following the recommendations outlined in Chapter 4 cannot be stressed enough. Weight control can decrease excess fat around the middle, lower insulin resistance, and lower blood pressure. A low-fat, high-fiber diet with a low glycemic index reduces the likelihood of developing metabolic syndrome through its effects on insulin resistance, weight control, and lipid levels. It also lowers markers of blood vessel inflammation. Inflammatory changes in blood vessels are known to have a key role in the development of cardiovascular disease. Engaging in regular, moderate-intensity exercise can improve your LDL and HDL levels, regardless of whether you lose a significant amount of weight as a result. This effect is probably related to exercise improving insulin resistance.

**Lipid Levels.**  Monitoring your lipid levels and promptly and aggressively treating abnormal levels is essential. Even slightly abnormal levels increase a woman's risk for having a heart attack. Elevated LDL and triglycerides are treated first with diet, by lowering fat intake and increasing fiber intake. If diet is not successful then medication is called for.

Raising low HDL levels is more difficult than lowering high LDL and triglyceride levels. Exercise is the most effective way to elevate your HDL levels. Diet has only a limited effect; a low-fat diet that includes foods containing omega-3 fatty acids is considered the most effective diet for raising HDL levels. Salmon is

## Medications to Lower Cholesterol

A number of medications are available to lower LDL and triglyceride levels. The most common types are statins, such as Lipitor, and fibrates, such as Tricor. Some medications are more effective at lowering LDLs, and others are better at lowering triglycerides. Your provider will choose the best one or a combination of both, on the basis of your blood test results.

one of the best sources of omega-3 fatty acids. The judicious consumption of alcohol (one or two drinks a day) also increases HDL levels. No medications are specifically designed to raise HDL levels, but fibrate drugs, a type of anticholesterol medication, have been found to have a positive effect. All of these measures will result in only a modest increase in HDL levels, but even a modest increase helps decrease cardiovascular risk, especially when combined with lower LDL levels.

**Blood Pressure.** You need to monitor your blood pressure. Checking it once or twice a year is sufficient if your blood pressure is well within the normal range. The normal range for the top number, called the systolic pressure, is 90 to 120; for the bottom number, the diastolic, it's 60 to 80. If either number starts creeping above its normal upper limit you need to take action. The first course of action is—you guessed it—to make lifestyle changes. Weight loss, exercise, and dietary changes often are all you need to keep your blood pressure where you want it. Lower your salt intake, limit alcohol to one drink a day, and avoid caffeine, along with making the dietary changes outlined in Chapter 4. Getting adequate sleep (seven to eight hours a night) and managing stress are also important in controlling blood pressure. This is where alternative therapies such as yoga, meditation, deep breathing exercises, and biofeedback can make a difference. If your blood pressure is consistently above 140/90 mm Hg despite lifestyle changes you will need to start medication.

*What Nurses Know...*

*A number of factors can raise your blood pressure temporarily. A stressful event, recent exercise, a sleepless night, or certain medications such as over-the-counter cold medicines can produce a single high reading. Some people have white-coat syndrome, a condition where just being in their health provider's office raises their blood pressure. If your blood pressure is high it should be checked on two or three occasions before you're diagnosed with hypertension.*

**Tobacco Use.** If you are a smoker, quit. Smoking triples your risk of dying of heart disease. Smoking triples your risk of developing diabetes. And smoking quadruples your risk of developing metabolic syndrome. Now multiply all those together and add in the increased risks associated with PCOS. The bottom line is that if you want to live a healthy life, you have to quit smoking.

Tobacco is highly addictive and quitting won't be easy, but there is no other single thing you can do that will have as much impact on your overall health. If you are ready to quit but are finding it difficult, talk to your provider about trying the medication bupropion, sold as Zyban or Wellbutrin. It is an antidepressant that for unknown reasons has been found to decrease the desire to smoke in people who want to quit. Nicotine patches can help you overcome the physical dependence on nicotine; they can be used alone or in combination with bupropion.

**Medication Adherence.** Consistently taking all the medications that you have been prescribed to treat PCOS is an important factor in decreasing the risk of diabetes and cardiovascular disease. Breaking the cycle of high androgen levels and insulin resistance helps reverse the risk of developing each of the characteristics of

• • • • • • • • • • • • • • • • • • • • • • • • • • •

## A Diabetes Primer

Diabetes mellitus is the full name of the condition commonly referred to simply as diabetes. (Another form of diabetes, diabetes insipidus, is a completely different disorder that has nothing to do with carbohydrate metabolism.) In the United States 8 percent of the population have diabetes mellitus. There are two types of diabetes mellitus: type I and type II. Type I used to be called juvenile diabetes because it usually starts in childhood or young adulthood. People with type I diabetes don't produce any insulin, so they need insulin injections to metabolize carbohydrates and control their blood sugar. Type II diabetes used to be known as late- or adult-onset diabetes because it usually first affects people in middle adulthood. With type II diabetes, either people don't produce enough insulin or their body tissues don't use insulin effectively. People with type II diabetes may be insulin dependent or non–insulin dependent, depending on whether their blood glucose can be controlled with diet and antidiabetic drugs or must be controlled with insulin injections. Diabetes mellitus is a leading cause of heart disease, stroke, kidney failure, adult blindness, and amputation of a foot or lower leg not related to trauma. It is the seventh leading cause of death overall.

metabolic syndrome. Maintaining stable glucose levels can delay or prevent the development of impaired glucose tolerance and the progression to diabetes.

### OBSTRUCTIVE SLEEP APNEA

Women with PCOS have higher rates of obstructive sleep apnea (OSA), a condition in which a person repeatedly stops breathing briefly during sleep. A person with OSA usually exhibits a pattern of loud snoring interrupted by periods of silence when breathing stops briefly, then inhalation with a gasp and loud snort when breathing resumes and snoring starts in again. This pattern repeats throughout the night—as few as 10 times or as many as 100 times.

OSA is caused by an obstructed airway. Normally during sleep the muscles of the throat relax but the upper throat stays open enough to allow airflow into the lungs. In OSA the upper part of the throat closes off completely or almost completely, blocking air from getting to the lungs and causing a brief spell of stalled breathing. The person makes a sudden attempt to breathe (the gasp and snort), awakening slightly each time.

People with OSA are not aware of the apnea or the sleep disruption that accompanies it. If you wake up every morning feeling like you had too late a night when you didn't or find yourself unusually sleepy during the day, you may have OSA. Talk to your provider about having a sleep study done.

Obesity is a reversible cause of OSA, and often losing weight will correct the problem. But there are other causes, such as a certain mouth or jaw shape or a narrow airway, for which other treatment options need to be pursued. And it appears that the incidence of OSA is increased among women with PCOS regardless of their weight.

Continuous positive airway pressure is the first-line treatment for OSA when weight loss doesn't work. A device delivers air under slight pressure through a mask you wear over your nose during sleep. The increased pressure keeps the throat muscles open.

Talk to your provider about treatment options if you've been diagnosed with OSA. Avoid alcohol, sleeping medications, and sedatives; they will worsen apnea.

⦁ ⦁ ⦁ ⦁ ⦁ ⦁ ⦁ ⦁ ⦁ ⦁ ⦁ ⦁ ⦁ ⦁ ⦁ ⦁ ⦁ ⦁ ⦁ ⦁ ⦁ ⦁ ⦁ ⦁ ⦁ ⦁ ⦁ ⦁

## Signs and Symptoms of OSA

If someone shares your sleeping space ask them whether they have observed the first three symptoms below, as you will not be aware of them. If you sleep alone and suspect on the basis of other symptoms that you may have OSA talk to your provider about having a sleep study done.

⦁ Loud snoring
⦁ Periods of apnea during sleep
⦁ Restless sleep
⦁ Abnormal daytime sleepiness
⦁ Waking up feeling tired
⦁ Morning headaches
⦁ Lethargy
⦁ Poor concentration

Don't ignore OSA. It is dangerous if left untreated. It can result in heart arrhythmias, high blood pressure, and stroke. Sleep deprivation can lead you to fall asleep in situations that put you at risk—behind the wheel of a car, for example. People with OSA have three times as many automobile accidents as those without the condition. And OSA increases your risk for heart disease, adding to all the other factors that increase this risk for a woman with PCOS.

## PCOS and Cancer

Women with PCOS are thought to be at greater risk for developing endometrial cancer. You may have read that there is also an increased risk of breast and ovarian cancer, but currently there is no evidence to support this. Endometrial cancer is the most common invasive gynecological cancer in the United States today. The prognosis is excellent when it is caught in the early stages. Some evidence suggests that premenopausal women with PCOS have an increased risk of endometrial cancer, although it's not conclusive and the true incidence of endometrial cancer in women with PCOS is unknown. Risk factors for endometrial cancer include obesity, never having been pregnant, infertility, diabetes, and hypertension—all factors common to PCOS. The most significant risk, however, is persistent estrogen exposure that's not moderated by progesterone, which occurs when you don't ovulate regularly.

Recall from Chapter 1 that ovulation starts the premenstrual phase of your menstrual cycle, leading to the drop-off in progesterone secretion that signals the endometrium to slough off. Chronic anovulation means that the endometrium continues to grow in response to estrogen that is "unopposed" by progesterone. This results in a condition called endometrial hyperplasia, an overgrowth of the cells and tissue of the endometrium. When endometrial hyperplasia persists some of the cells may become abnormal, or atypical, resulting in a condition called atypical hyperplasia. Atypical hyperplasia is a precursor to cancer. It is thought that high levels of insulin in the blood may also contribute to the increased risk of endometrial cancer in women with PCOS, through insulin's effect on endometrial cell growth.

The fewer periods you have, the greater the risk that you will develop endometrial hyperplasia and atypical hyperplasia. Therefore, the mainstay of prevention is the use of either combination OCPs or progesterone pills to induce withdrawal bleeding. Combination OCPs contain both estrogen and progesterone and regulate your menstrual cycle by inducing regular monthly withdrawal bleeding (we call this a "period," but the period you have every month while on OCPs is actually withdrawal bleeding). OCPs have the added benefits of suppressing androgen production and lowering the risk of endometrial and ovarian cancer.

The periodic use of progesterone medications also induces withdrawal bleeding. A nonandrogenic progesterone, either Provera or Prometrium, is prescribed for 10 days. About three to seven days after you stop the progesterone (the "withdrawal") you will begin to bleed. The duration and amount of bleeding depend on how built up the endometrial tissue is. If you don't bleed at all or bleeding continues for more than seven days or you are soaking a sanitary pad every hour, you need to notify your doctor. There is no hard-and-fast rule about how often withdrawal bleeding should occur, but experts generally agree that you should have a withdrawal bleed at least every three months. This will prevent endometrial hyperplasia and guard against the withdrawal bleeding being too prolonged or heavy.

The other situation that requires withdrawal bleeding is when the endometrium is thicker than 10 mm, as measured using ultrasound. Your provider should do a follow-up ultrasound after the withdrawal bleed to make sure the endometrium has shed. If it hasn't, a biopsy or a dilatation and curettage (D&C) may be required.

There are no early signs of endometrial cancer, so you must keep track of your periods and any withdrawal bleeding you have. Late symptoms can include unusual vaginal bleeding or discharge, difficulty urinating, pain with sexual intercourse, and

## Dilatation and Curettage

The D&C procedure is performed by a gynecologist, either in the outpatient setting of the hospital or in the physician's office. You may be given local anesthesia or general anesthesia for the procedure.

The doctor dilates (opens) the cervix by inserting progressively larger probes into the cervical opening. Once the cervix is sufficiently dilated, an instrument called a curette is passed through and used to scrape the endometrial tissue from the walls of the uterus.

After the procedure you may experience some lower abdominal cramping and spotting. You should not have sexual intercourse or use tampons or douche for a week after the procedure. If you have heavy bleeding, fever, abdominal pain, or a foul-smelling discharge notify your physician right away.

pain in the pelvic area. Pap smears do not screen for endometrial cancer, only cervical cancer. Endometrial cancer usually has an excellent prognosis in premenopausal women, but nothing beats prevention.

## Resources

### American Cancer Society
For general information about cancer prevention go to the Health Information Seekers link under the heading "I need information for..."

### American Diabetes Association
This organization provides comprehensive information about diabetes for professionals and the general public. Information about type I and type II diabetes, prevention, and symptoms can be found under the heading "Diabetes Basics."
http://www.diabetes.org/

### American Heart Association
This well-known organization also provides comprehensive information for professionals and the general public on their

Web site. It includes information on metabolic syndrome as well as heart disease. The "Healthy Lifestyle" link has information on how to live a heart-healthy life and a section devoted specifically to women.
http://www.americanheart.org

### Medline Plus
You can find information on metabolic syndrome and heart disease under the "Health Topics" heading. It also has links to numerous other resources for each condition.
http://www.nlm.nih.gov/medlineplus/medlineplus.html

### National Heart Lung and Blood Institute
This is a branch of the National Institutes for Health. On their Web site under the "Public" heading you can find extensive information about both metabolic syndrome and heart disease. They also have a section specific to women.
http://www.nhlbi.nih.gov/index.htm

### National Research Center for Women and Families
This site gives you easy-to-understand information on the latest research on cancer as well as other topics important to women.
http://www.center4research.org

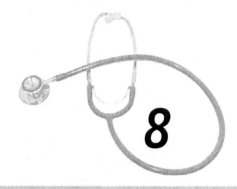

# 8

# Mental Health

*I'm constantly fighting it [PCOS]. The constant struggle makes it hard to just be happy and stay on top of your game twenty-four/ seven. Sometimes you can't deal with it. You feel so bad; the hormones are so out of whack. You don't want to get up out of bed. You don't want to face it. But I'm a strong person. I'm going to push on, push forward.   STEPHANIE*

*People don't understand the psychological stuff that goes with it, the depression and anger. I get so angry over nothing. Some days I'm happy-go-lucky, everything is fine, and other days I'm just so depressed or enraged for no reason whatsoever. Every little thing is a struggle. I hate to be the person to blame things on PCOS; I don't want to use it as an excuse. But it's not an excuse! It's the reason why I feel this way.   AMY*

PCOS is associated with many outward signs: the acne, the excessive hair growth, the struggle with weight control. These are distressing, but an invisible side of PCOS that many women face can be even more difficult: the mental and emotional effects. If you are experiencing depression, anxiety, anger, chronic fatigue, or low self-esteem, you are not alone.

Most women with PCOS don't have debilitating psychological symptoms. You are able to go through your day doing all the normal things people do. But you may have to work harder at staying happy, or you may not really enjoy life much, or your enjoyment may be frequently interrupted by anger, sadness, irritability, or feeling overwhelmed. You may have a short temper that sometimes feels out of your control. All this might affect your relationships, your love life, your job, and your plans for the future. The bottom line is that the invisible side of PCOS most certainly affects your quality of life, whether you are aware of it or not.

PCOS should not turn your life into an endurance test. There are ways to manage the emotional fallout.

## Changing Your Perspective

If you often wish you could be "normal" you are not alone. Most women with PCOS at some point think of themselves as different from "normal" women. Many even say they feel like "freaks."

You are not a freak—no more than a woman with diabetes or asthma or a heart murmur is a freak. It is reasonable to want to feel attractive. We all want that. No one should tell you that you're being silly because you're unhappy with being overweight or you're self-conscious about the hair on your face. Do not mistake symptoms of a disorder for signs of abnormality; you are a normal woman who struggles with the symptoms of an endocrine disorder. **You are not your symptoms.**

Many women with PCOS report a sense of being "less of a woman" or "not a real woman" because of their symptoms. This feeling can be sparked by the frequent description of the disorder as simply having too many male hormones rather than as the complex endocrine and metabolic disorder it is. It is also related to symptoms, such as excess hair growth, that make it even harder than usual to live up to society's standards for feminine beauty. Infertility is another cause; motherhood is still considered by many to be a woman's primary role in life, and not fulfilling that role can make you feel like a failure as a woman.

But what does it mean to be feminine anyway? The dictionary defines feminine as "pertaining to a woman" or "having qualities attributed to women." That leaves it pretty wide open, which is where society steps in. Remember who dominated society until recently…that's right: men. Current definitions of femininity derive from the qualities men decided women should have. Those qualities included not being too smart or too independent. They included modesty and sexual reserve. Being feminine meant being weak and soft. This is changing; today women are strong, independent, and smart, and they enjoy their sexuality. No one has a patent on femininity. Some women feel feminine when they're dressed a certain way, whether in ruffles and lace or a pinstriped power suit. Some find femininity in fragrances or jewelry; others in the sweat that follows a 10-mile run. Some find it in the act of loving a child or caring for an elderly parent. Some find it in a steamy night of lovemaking. Wherever you find it, femininity is an essence within you. It may be brought out by certain things, but it is not contained in those things.

## Depression and Anxiety

### DEPRESSION

Women with PCOS are at a greater risk for depression and anxiety, regardless of their other symptoms. This means that depression or anxiety is not necessarily the result of your being down about constantly dealing with such symptoms as obesity or infertility, and your chance of being depressed is not related to how bad your other symptoms are. Why woman with PCOS have an increased risk of depression is not known. An increased risk of depression is also associated with another condition common among women with PCOS: diabetes. But the link between depression and diabetes is not understood either.

We can all probably think of a time when we have complained about being "depressed," feeling down while going through a tough patch. After a few days, we pick ourselves up and move on. The problem comes when we can't pick ourselves up, when we can't move on. Feelings of sadness and hopelessness linger or worsen. Just getting through the day can become a monumental struggle.

Depression is a real illness. It is not laziness or weakness or just feeling sorry for yourself. Do not let anyone tell you differently. You can't just snap out of it; you need help. Depression interferes with your ability to enjoy life and can take away your ability to function normally. It affects your job, your relationships, and your physical health. At its worst it can make you feel

● ● ● ● ● ● ● ● ● ● ● ● ● ● ● ● ● ● ● ● ● ● ● ● ● ● ● ●

## Signs and Symptoms of Depression

Symptoms of depression range from vague feelings of unhappiness that don't go away to constant crying for no reason. If you have any of the following symptoms for two weeks or more talk to your health care provider and look into counseling:

- Loss of interest in normal activities
- Feeling sad or down
- Feeling hopeless or worthless
- Crying for no reason
- Sleeping problems
- Difficulty focusing or concentrating
- Difficulty making decisions
- Irritability
- Restlessness
- Unusual fatigue or weakness
- Loss of interest in sex
- Unintentional weight loss
- Unexplained weight gain
- Unexplained physical symptoms such as back pain, headaches, or no appetite

If you have thoughts of hurting yourself get help immediately. If you find yourself taking chances with your safety—driving dangerously, overmedicating yourself, drinking excessively—get help immediately.

like you no longer want to live. But help is available. Counseling and medication can be effective for even the worst depression and in two or three weeks have you feeling much better.

## ANXIETY

It is natural to feel anxious in certain situations, and normal anxiety can be a good thing. It's what primes athletes or actors to perform at their best; it pushes us to study for a test, prepare well for an important event, or be cautious when faced with risk. Anxiety becomes a problem when it is constant or severe and interferes with our ability to function normally. Anxiety that has no specific cause is called free-floating or generalized anxiety disorder. Stress does not cause generalized anxiety disorder, but it can worsen it. Certainly the stress of dealing with a chronic illness such as PCOS can worsen anxiety.

Depression and anxiety often go hand in hand. Effective treatment is available for both. The biggest barrier to getting treatment is the stigma associated with being diagnosed with a "mental illness." The first step to feeling better is accepting that these emotional symptoms are exactly that—symptoms—and should be treated as such. They do not carry any moral judgment about your character, any more than irregular periods or insulin resistance does. Seeking treatment is the next step, whether through counseling, CAM, medication, or some combination of the three.

## What Nurses Know...

You deserve a happy life. Don't wait for anxiety or depression to be severe before you seek help. There is nothing admirable or character building about needless suffering. There is no reason to struggle every day with depression or anxiety, to allow it to limit your life, when effective and safe treatment is available.

## COUNSELING

Counseling has many benefits. It gives you a safe place to vent frustrations, fears, grief, and all the other difficult emotions that accompany a chronic illness. It can help you discover coping mechanisms to deal with the emotional fallout of PCOS.

Finding the right counselor is essential. Start by asking your endocrinologist or primary care provider for recommendations. If you belong to a support group check with other women in the group. Talk to friends and family members you trust; you'd be surprised how many people are getting therapy today. Contact a counseling center in your area for information on local therapists.

Check the credentials of any counselor you are considering; it is important that you work with someone with the necessary educational preparation and experience. Ask potential therapists about their training and experience, including the certifications they hold, how long they've been in practice, and whether they have treated clients with problems similar to yours.

Give yourself some time to find the right person. Don't settle on the first counselor you see. Plan on making a number of phone calls and a few visits to different counselors before deciding. It's not unusual to feel nervous with someone at first, but after that if you don't feel you can talk easily and safely about what is bothering you the most, you need to find another counselor. Therapy with the wrong counselor is not only ineffective; it can be harmful.

• • • • • • • • • • • • • • • • • • • • • • • • • • • •

## Money Matters

Check your health insurance policy before your first appointment. Most policies cover counseling services to some extent, but you may need to take specific steps to get visits paid for. Some policies require you to notify the health insurance company before you start or cover services only if you see certain therapists.

If you don't have health insurance ask whether the therapist offers a sliding fee scale, where payment is based on your income level: the lower your income, the less you pay. Check around before seeing someone who doesn't offer this; there is certain to be a clinic or individual therapist in your area that does.

Counselors come in all shapes and sizes, with all kinds of initials after their names. The most common types and qualifications are listed here:

- A psychiatrist (MD) is a medical doctor who spent four years of residency specializing in psychiatry. Psychiatrists can prescribe medications. They usually work with people who have mental illness that requires intensive therapy or complex medication management.
- A doctor of psychology (PsyD) has a doctorate degree in psychology and focuses on clinical work such as therapy. Doctors of psychology cannot prescribe medications.
- A doctor of philosophy (PhD) has a doctorate degree that prepares him or her to do research and therapy. Doctors of philosophy cannot prescribe medications.
- A social worker (MSW) has a master's degree in social work and is prepared to do therapy with attention to the social and cultural context of the individual or family. A social worker cannot prescribe medications.
- A psychiatric or mental health nurse practitioner (NP) is a nurse with an advanced practice degree, either a master's or doctorate, that prepares him or her to do therapy. A nurse practitioner can prescribe medications.

Therapists who cannot prescribe medications will liaise with your primary care provider if medications are needed. Even though they are not licensed to prescribe, they are usually well informed about the different medication options. If your therapist does prescribe medications, make sure it is in consultation with your primary care provider and that everyone has an updated list of the medications you're on.

## COMPLEMENTARY AND ALTERNATIVE MEDICINE

A number of complementary and alternative therapies are used to treat depression and anxiety. Many people find them helpful, though there is little scientific evidence to support their use.

## What Nurses Know...

Finding the right counselor is the key to successful counseling. You must feel comfortable with your counselor and be able to talk easily after the first couple of visits. After the first couple of visits ask yourself these questions:

- Do I trust this person?
- Do I have a good rapport with this person?
- Did I feel like this person is judging me in any way?
- Do I feel like they get it?
- How do I feel as the time for a visit nears?
- How do I feel when I leave?

If any of your answers are unsatisfactory, find another counselor.

You must be as careful in choosing a CAM treatment as you are when choosing traditional treatments. This is especially true of supplements and herbal medicine, which can have bad side effects or interact with other drugs you are taking or with each other. Also, think carefully before opting for a CAM treatment over traditional medication. Declining a treatment that has been proven to work for one that hasn't may mean you do not reach the optimum level of health possible and could even jeopardize your future health.

The following are safe CAM therapies you may want to try:

- Acupuncture is a traditional Chinese treatment that uses needles in certain spots on the body to restore the balance of yin and yang forces. It is safe, and some scientific evidence exists to support its use in depression and anxiety. It sounds painful, but it's not; people say it's a relaxing and pleasant experience.

- Aromatherapy uses concentrated essential oils, which may be applied directly to the skin, used in the bath, or diffused into the air. Aromatherapy is relaxing; it can help relieve stress and may lessen anxiety. It may improve your mood, but it is not effective for moderate or severe depression.
- Light therapy uses prolonged exposure to bright light of a specific wavelength to relieve depression. It is very effective for winter depression, also known as seasonal affective disorder, and recent studies suggest that it is also helpful for nonseasonal depression.
- Relaxation techniques include meditation, guided imagery, and progressive muscle relaxation. They are used to create a state of calm focus and relaxation and can help relieve stress and anxiety. Yoga and tai chi are other relaxation approaches that many people have used successfully.
- Music therapy has been shown to be very effective at relieving stress, anxiety, and depression. Listening to music and making music yourself both work. The type of music depends on what you enjoy, though soothing sounds are usually best if you are stressed or anxious. Engaging a professional music therapist may help get you started, but it's not necessary.

**Exercise.** You may not think of exercise as a treatment, but it is an effective way to lessen the symptoms of depression and anxiety. Studies have shown that 30 minutes of exercise a day can make a big difference. It works in a number of ways: it increases your self-esteem, relaxes tense muscles, distracts you from focusing on problems, raises endorphin levels in your blood, and lowers levels of the stress hormone cortisol. And remember that exercise has numerous other positive effects on PCOS symptoms.

**Herbs.** A number of herbs have been used to treat depression and anxiety, including kava (*Piper methysticum*), St. John's wort (*Hypericum perforatum*), and valerian (*Valeriana officinalis*). It is a good idea to talk with your provider before starting any herb or supplement and a must if you are taking any medications.

Kava is used to treat anxiety, and many studies have found it to be effective. It has been shown to relieve anxiety and improve sleep without affecting clarity of thought in the way some sedatives can. The problem is that it has also been shown to cause severe liver disease, including liver failure. In fact, some countries, including the United Kingdom, have banned its use. In the United States the FDA has issued an advisory stating that people with liver disease should contact their physician before taking any product that contains kava.

St. John's wort has been shown to be effective as a treatment for mild to moderate depression. Some studies have shown it to be as effective as SSRIs, the most commonly prescribed antidepressant medications. St. John's wort is relatively safe; the most common

## What Nurses Know...

Do not take a product containing kava if any of the following statements fits you:

- You have a history of alcohol abuse.
- You have a history of liver problems.
- You have a history of kidney problems.
- You have a bleeding disorder.
- You are pregnant, trying to get pregnant, or nursing.
- You have had surgery within the past two weeks.

If you are taking kava and have any of the following side effects report them to your provider right away:

- Yellowing of the skin (jaundice)
- Unusual fatigue
- Abdominal pain
- Loss of appetite
- Nausea or vomiting
- Joint pain

side effects are stomach upset, rash, headache, and dizziness. However, you still need to take it under the supervision of your provider: it can interact with numerous other medications and, more importantly, you should not try to treat depression by yourself. You should involve a professional who can help you through the depression and monitor your progress. Do not take St. John's wort if you are pregnant, trying to get pregnant, or nursing.

Valerian has been used for a long time to treat sleep problems and anxiety. There is very little research on its effectiveness, however. A few studies have shown it to be helpful for insomnia. It can cause headaches, dizziness, and upset stomach, and sometimes you may wake up feeling tired the morning after taking it.

Other herbs used for depression and anxiety include ginkgo (*Ginkgo biloba*), passionflower (*Passiflora incarnata*), ginger (*Zingiber officinale*), and chamomile (*Matricaria chamomilla*). Little is known about their effectiveness, and, as with all herbs and supplements, they should be used under the supervision of your provider.

**Supplements.** A number of dietary supplements are recommended for someone being treated for depression or anxiety. This is primarily because a deficiency in any of them has been linked to a higher risk of depression and anxiety. It can also be because stress increases your body's need for them. These supplements include omega-3 fatty acids, B-complex vitamins, especially folate, vitamin C, vitamin D, magnesium, calcium, iron, and manganese. Taking a daily multivitamin that includes these vitamins and minerals may improve your mood and help you handle the stresses of living with PCOS.

• • • • • • • • • • • • • • • • • • • • • • • • • •

## Alert

Do not use kava, St. John's wort, or valerian with other antidepressant or antianxiety medications. This can lead to a dangerous overdose.

Kava, St. John's wort, and valerian interact with a number of other medications, so be sure to check with your provider before taking them.

## MEDICATIONS

Medication can help if you are struggling with depression and anxiety and other measures have not helped. The most commonly used antidepressants are SSRIs and serotonin and norepinephrine reuptake inhibitors (SNRIs). These medications can be very effective and have few side effects when used appropriately. The most commonly prescribed antianxiety medications are the SSRIs and SNRIs, benzodiazepines, and buspirone.

It is important to find the right drug and the right dosage for you. Antidepressant and antianxiety medications are not meant to make you feel life is wonderful all the time, nor are they meant to make you numb. They are intended to take the edge off the emotional extremes that disrupt and limit your life. They don't make everything better, but they do help you deal better with what comes your way. They also relieve anxiety and panic attacks.

> There's a lot of moodiness but I don't want to take antidepressants. I do have severe sleep problems though—insomnia. I take a milligram of Xanax at bedtime if I can't fall asleep, not all the time. It helps a lot.  STEPHANIE

## What Nurses Know...

There are many SSRI and SNRI medications out there, and sometimes it takes trial and error to find the right one and the right dose for you. If one drug doesn't work or the side effects bother you, try a different one, or ask about starting at a lower dose and slowly increasing the dose as your body adjusts to the medication.

Don't give up on the first try; used correctly, SSRIs and SNRIs can make a real difference. They should not, however, have you walking around in la-la land.

*I was on Effexor for a while but I didn't like it. Yeah, I didn't feel so angry anymore—but I didn't feel anything else either. I don't want to walk around not feeling anything. Sometimes though I feel like I need to go back on it. Maybe if I find someone who's good, a good endocrinologist, they'll change the dose or try something else that will work better. I'd go back on something then.*   AMY

**SSRIs and SNRIs.**   SSRIs and SNRIs act on chemicals in the brain to relieve depression and anxiety. They are not habit forming. It usually takes at least two to three weeks to feel better after you start taking them, though some people report feeling better much earlier. Continue your medication after you start feeling better; you are probably feeling better *because* of the medication. Talk to your counselor and other providers before deciding to stop taking the medication. You must stop the medication gradually or you will get withdrawal symptoms. Although SSRIs are not addictive, they can cause such symptoms as dizziness, headache, nausea, and diarrhea when they are stopped, especially if they are stopped abruptly.

**Benzodiazepines.**   Benzodiazepines are the medications commonly known as sedatives. Whereas SSRIs need time to build up to a certain level and then control symptoms by maintaining that steady level in your system, benzodiazepines work immediately and are used on an as-needed basis. They are habit forming, though, and you can build up a tolerance over time, so they generally should not be used daily or for extended periods. If you have ever had problems with addiction you should try SSRIs instead. Otherwise benzodiazepines are a good choice if you need to take something for anxiety only once in a while or to relieve anxiety attacks or panic attacks. Do not use benzodiazepines if you are pregnant, trying to get pregnant, or nursing.

### BUSPIRONE
Buspirone (Buspar) is an antianxiety medication that may be prescribed to treat anxiety if SSRIs are not effective or are not

## Alert

Some studies indicate that SSRIs and SNRIs may increase the risk of suicide in people younger than 25. If you are under 25 and taking an SSRI or SNRI, ensure close follow-up with your provider throughout the time you are on the medication but especially in the first few weeks. Set up a weekly follow-up visit and phone checks with the nurse in between for the first month.

No matter what your age, make sure that you follow up closely with your provider during the first two weeks after starting an antidepressant. This is when the risk of suicide is highest, which is thought to be because people have improved enough to have the energy to make a suicide attempt but not enough to overcome the depressed mood.

### SSRIs and SNRIs

The more common side effects of SSRI and SNRI medications include drowsiness, dizziness, headache, sleep problems, vivid and strange dreams, apathy, changes in appetite, weight loss or gain, and sexual problems. Many people find that if they can hold out a couple of weeks the side effects improve. This is only for mild or moderate side effects, however. You should not continue a medication with intolerable side effects; there are other options.

The following drugs are SSRIs:

- Citalopram (Celexa)
- Escitalopram (Lexapro)
- Fluoxetine (Prozac)
- Fluvoxamine (Luvox)
- Paroxetine (Paxil)
- Sertraline (Zoloft)

The following drugs are SNRIs:

- Duloxetine (Cymbalta)
- Venlafaxine (Effexor)

tolerated. It is also often used as an additional medication for anxiety when SSRI therapy alone is not adequately relieving symptoms. It differs from the benzodiazepines in that it does not act immediately, taking up to two weeks to work, and it does not cause sedation. It can cause drowsiness however, so you need to

## Benzodiazepines

The most common side effects of benzodiazepines are drowsiness, constipation, and nausea. Benzodiazepines can be addictive and are usually prescribed only for short-term use. The following drugs are benzodiazepines:

- Alprazolam (Xanax)
- Clonazepam (Klonopin)
- Diazepam (Valium)
- Lorazepam (Ativan)

be careful until you see how it affects you. You should not drink alcohol while taking buspirone because alcohol will increase the occurrence of side effects, particularly dizziness, and may decrease the effectiveness of the medication. You should also not eat grapefruit or drink grapefruit juice while taking buspirone as it changes the way the drug is metabolized in a way that causes a dangerous increase in the amount of the drug in your system. (Grapefruit can do this with a number of medications so you should always ask your health care provider about it when starting a new medication.)

## Resources

### American Association of Pastoral Counselors
This association supports psychological services that are grounded in theology and spirituality. The Web site has a referral directory to find certified pastoral counselors.
www.aapc.org/

### American Psychological Association
The Web site for this professional organization offers consumer information on mind/body health including dealing with stress and anger.
www.apa.org/helpcenter/index.aspx

### MedlinePlus: Mental Health
Offers comprehensive information on mental health as well as numerous links to other resources.
www.nlm.nih.gov/medlineplus/mentalhealth.html

### Mental Health America
This Web site offers extensive information on mental health that is searchable by audience, issue, or disorders and treatment.
www.nmha.org/

### National Association of Social Workers
*This Web site maintains a listing of clinical social workers that have met national certification standards.*
www.naswdc.org/

### National Mental Health Information Center
Comprehensive information from the U.S. Department of Health and Human Services.
http://mentalhealth.samhsa.gov/

### Psychology Today
*User-friendly site geared to consumers with engaging articles and all kinds of*
www.psychologytoday.com/

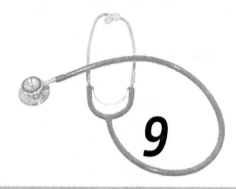

*9*

# Becoming a Family

*I've been trying to have a baby for the last five years. I've been on Clomid three times. I thought once I started eating better, and then after I lost the weight, that my blood chemistry would change and things would start working correctly. I was so discouraged when I didn't start ovulating. I went for a third try of Clomid. I thought for sure it's going to happen this time. This last time I was on Clomid for two months. A couple of follicles started to enlarge but they didn't get big enough. So then I started injections. But then all of a sudden I had a lot of blood in my urine so we had to halt everything, again!*

*I'm mentally and physically exhausted and I don't know who to talk to. Generally I find that on Web sites or support groups for infertility, you don't find a lot of women with PCOS. So I don't really find them helpful; they don't have the same problems. I feel like I'm going through this alone. I have women friends who are supportive; they're behind me one hundred percent. But they're basically ears, no advice really.*

*Sometimes I just want to give up completely on trying to have a baby. My friends say, "Don't give up! Don't give up!" I'm kind of ready to be done with it. I think I'll keep trying until I'm thirty-five. That's when all the books say your chances of getting pregnant decrease so much and chances of birth defects go up and there's more risks. I don't want in vitro. Anyway it's not an option; it's just way too expensive.*

*Everything is so expensive. You can't get it covered on insurance if it's fertility treatments. And as soon as you say you want to have a baby they stop paying for other things too. You go from a woman with PCOS to a woman wanting fertility.*

*I think if my husband was your average person I probably still wouldn't be married. He's always made me feel as comfortable as possible. I think it would change me if I had a baby, but it wouldn't change our marriage.*

*We've thought about adoption but I don't know. I think if I don't get pregnant there's a reason. We're going to do the best we can and if it doesn't happen…*

*So, now what? I guess I'm still trying to figure out where I'm going to go from here.  STEPHANIE*

*I was tired all the time and had gained a lot of weight, so I went to the doctor. He said either you're pregnant or you're depressed and eating too much. He had me fill out a questionnaire and gave me some medication and told me to stop eating so much. He never did a pregnancy test. I started taking the Effexor and felt better after a couple of weeks, so I didn't think much more about it. My boyfriend and I had broken up months ago, so I wasn't even having sex. Pregnancy was the last thing on my mind.*

*Months later I woke up with really bad stomach pain. I thought a cyst had burst; that's what it felt like. I worked all day in terrible pain. When I got home I went right to bed. When my mom asked me if there was any chance I could be pregnant I got really mad and upset. How could she even ask me that! I have PCOS–I'm not supposed to even be able to get pregnant! She ran to the store to buy a pregnancy test and…it was positive.*

*I started flipping out. I didn't believe it. I said it must be positive because my hormones are all messed up with the PCOS. In the ER my mom told the nurse, "I think my daughter's in labor." I started yelling, "I am not! How dare you!" They took me upstairs and hooked me up to the monitor. I heard a noise and asked the nurse what it was. She said, "That's your baby's heartbeat."*

*I was in shock. I felt numb and terrified. I remember thinking, "If he comes out messed up in any way…" All those months I had been partying with friends, taking medications that are bad for pregnancy. I was praying he would come out healthy.*

*And he did. I needed a C-section but he was fine. I was in shock for a couple of months. Literally overnight I went from being a carefree twenty-one-year-old doing whatever, whenever, to a mother with a baby depending on me for everything. And I know people were judging me; they didn't believe I didn't know. They didn't understand that with PCOS a lot of symptoms are the same as being pregnant. No periods, the weight gain, being tired. For a while I was happiest when I was alone, just me and Ben.*

*It was after Ben was born that I realized I didn't have a clue what PCOS was, really. I hadn't taken my medication consistently or paid attention to my diet. I decided it was time to start paying attention.   AMY*


Having a family is one of the biggest challenges that women with PCOS face. Infertility is common because women with PCOS have problems with ovulation related to the hormonal changes associated with the disorder.

Problems aren't limited to getting pregnant. The symptoms of pregnancy can mirror those of PCOS and may go unnoticed, leading to lack of prenatal care. PCOS increases the risk of miscarriage and complications late in pregnancy such as gestational diabetes and preeclampsia. The rate of cesarean sections is also higher in women with PCOS.

The picture is not completely bleak, however. There are measures you can take to increase your chances of getting pregnant, staying pregnant, and safely giving birth to a healthy baby. The majority of women with PCOS who want to have a baby are successful. Like everything else, it begins with you: lifestyle changes are the first step, followed by fertility treatments.

## What Nurses Know...

Don't wait to get pregnant to start doing the right things for nurturing a developing baby. You may not even know you are pregnant in the first crucial weeks, when the most rapid development is happening. Begin at least a month ahead of time with the following steps:

- Start taking prenatal-strength multivitamins.
- Take at least 400 micrograms of folic acid daily.
- If you smoke, stop.
- Wean yourself off caffeine.
- Eat a healthy, balanced diet.
- Get as close as possible to a healthy BMI.
- Engage in moderate exercise. (If you are on fertility treatment, check with your provider first.)
- Review your medications with your provider to see whether any of them are harmful to a fetus and should be stopped while you're trying to get pregnant.

If you have been trying to get pregnant for a year without success, or for six months if you are 35 or older, then it is time to seek help. In the meantime you can take action to maximize your chance of getting pregnant and having a healthy pregnancy, starting with lifestyle changes.

One other important note. Do not assume that having PCOS means you are the cause of all your problems conceiving. One-third of cases of infertility are caused by problems in women, one-third by problems in men, and one-third by a combination of factors in both partners. Therefore it is vital that he is involved in the treatment and is tested at the beginning. Don't be surprised when your fertility specialist asks him to undergo a semen analysis. You don't want to go through months of expensive, emotionally draining treatment only to find out that all along his sperm count was too low for it ever to have worked.

## Stat Facts

- Infertility affects approximately 7.3 million women in the United States.
- Infertility affects between 10 and 20 percent of people of childbearing age.
- PCOS causes 75 percent of cases of infertility related to anovulation.
- Medication or surgery can be used to treat 85 to 90 percent of cases of infertility.

## Lifestyle Changes

The best thing you can do when you are trying to get pregnant is maintain a healthy weight. In Chapter 4 we talked about all the positive effects of weight loss and how important it is in managing PCOS. It is especially important if you are trying to conceive. Losing as little as 5 to 7 percent of your body weight can result in the resumption of ovulation, so weight loss is considered the first-line infertility treatment in any woman who is obese. And if you do pursue fertility treatments it has been found that obese women need higher doses of fertility drugs over a longer period for the treatments to work.

However, if you are older than 34 or have been trying to get pregnant for longer than a year and a half, some experts think that time may be more important than weight. In these situations your chances of a successful pregnancy may depend more on how soon you get started on infertility treatments than on how close you get to a healthy weight. You may not want to delay infertility treatments while you try to lose weight.

Weight loss has benefits beyond increasing your chance of getting pregnant. Obesity increases the risk of miscarriage, gestational diabetes, and preeclampsia whether you have PCOS or not. Starting a pregnancy at a healthy weight is best for you and your baby.

Exercise will help with weight control. However, you should avoid intense workouts. When you are on infertility treatments there may be times when you need to limit your activity, so check with your fertility specialist before exercising.

As discussed in Chapter 4, the best diet for women with PCOS is a low-fat, low-glycemic-index diet. This holds true when you are trying to conceive and during a pregnancy. You should also eat plenty of leafy green vegetables, high-fiber grains, protein, and foods high in vitamin C. Start taking a multivitamin with folic acid a month before you start trying to conceive. Folic acid reduces the risk of birth defects of the brain and spinal cord if you start taking it *before* pregnancy.

If you smoke, quit. It's that simple. Smoking interferes with your hormones, lowers your chances of conceiving, increases your chances of having a miscarriage, and is harmful to a developing baby.

The same is true for alcohol. Once you start trying to conceive you should not drink alcohol at all. Alcohol interferes with ovulation and decreases your chances of getting pregnant. Drinking during pregnancy has well-known serious effects on a developing baby.

## Infertility Treatments

### GETTING STARTED

Choosing to seek infertility treatment is a big decision. Treatment is costly, time consuming, and emotionally draining. You and your partner need to educate yourselves about the details of treatments and discuss them in advance. You must both be committed to the process. Before you begin treatment you should

## What Nurses Know...

Write down your feelings and your decisions before starting the treatment. Looking back at these notes will help you think clearly about things later, when you are feeling frustrated, exhausted, and unsure of how to proceed.

know where you're going with it. Decide now what types of treatments you want to try and how you will know it's time to stop. Is in vitro fertilization an option if other methods don't work, for example? How much money are you willing to spend?

The next step is to choose a fertility specialist. Some OB/GYN doctors treat infertility, but women with PCOS should see a reproductive endocrinologist from the start. A reproductive endocrinologist is an OB/GYN doctor who has undergone extensive additional training in treating infertility. He or she will be better prepared to deal with the complex hormonal factors in infertility related to PCOS.

## What Nurses Know...

Schedule consultations with a number of reproductive specialists before deciding which one to see. You want to find out the following information:

Are they board certified as a reproductive endocrinologist?
How long have they been treating infertility?
What is the full range of services they offer?
How much experience do they have of treating women with PCOS?
What are the success rates? What are the success rates for women with PCOS and for women your age?
What would your treatment plan be?
How much would the treatment cost?
What insurance plans do they accept?
Are long-term payments or other financing options available?
What are the office hours? Do they have evening or weekend hours?
Whom can you talk to when the office is closed?

Make sure you choose someone you are comfortable with. You will be discussing personal, intimate details with this person. Infertility treatments can be difficult and emotionally trying. You need someone who is responsive to your questions and concerns. You also need to think about location, as treatments may require frequent trips to the doctor's office. It is ideal if your reproductive endocrinologist works in a fertility clinic with a good support staff and access to the full range of reproductive technologies.

### FERTILITY TREATMENTS

Fertility treatments range from drugs to help you ovulate to advanced technologies such as in vitro fertilization. Before treatment is started a number of tests will be done. You will already have had many of these tests as part of your workup for PCOS, but if more than a few months have gone by your infertility specialist will probably repeat them.

- Blood tests for FSH, estradiol, prolactin, TSH, fasting glucose, hepatitis, syphilis, HIV, measles, chicken pox, and blood type
- Pelvic ultrasound
- Hysterosalpingogram, an x-ray to check for blockages that would prevent an egg from moving freely through the fallopian tubes into the uterus. The x-ray is taken while dye is injected through the vagina into the uterus.

Before starting treatment your fertility specialist may advise you to try timed intercourse. With this method you have intercourse every other day during the time you are most fertile—when you are ovulating. Many women keep track of when they are most fertile by measuring their basal body temperature every morning *before* getting out of bed. A woman's temperature rises slightly, by about half to one degree, immediately after she ovulates. After a few months of using this method, women can figure out when they're most likely to be ovulating. However, this method doesn't work for most women with PCOS because their

## Money Matters

The costs of fertility treatments may or may not be covered under your health insurance plan. In some states insurers are required by law to cover them, but in most states they are not. Before you start treatment check the regulations in your state. Call your health insurance office and talk to a representative (make sure you get the representative's name). Ask the following questions:

- Am I covered for infertility treatment under my current plan?
- If not, is there a rider I can purchase that would provide coverage?
- If I am covered, what are the benefits?
- Are there any restrictions?
- Am I covered for diagnostic tests? Treatment procedures? Drugs? (Ask about specific tests, procedures, and drugs.)
- Do I need a referral?
- Do I need precertification? If so, how long is it good for?
- What are the maximum allowable benefits? Does it go by calendar year or lifetime?
- Do I need to use specific specialists or reproductive centers?

cycles are so irregular. Another method of tracking ovulation, which may be more effective for women with PCOS, is a fertility test kit or monitor. These tests detect the rise in LH that happens just before ovulation, giving you advance notice. Unfortunately this method will not work for women with PCOS who always run high LH levels. And timing intercourse to coincide with ovulation will not work for women who do not ovulate at all.

The decision to start infertility treatments has been made. You've chosen your specialist and contacted your insurance company. You're ready to begin. Now what?

**Step 1: Clomiphene Citrate.**   The first-line medication for treatment of infertility in women with PCOS—and most women, in fact—is clomiphene citrate (Clomid) to induce ovulation. Clomiphene citrate has been used successfully to treat infertility since 1967, so it has a long and proven track record. It induces ovulation in 80 percent of women with PCOS, and about 45 percent of them conceive.

It is safe, easy to take (because it is a pill not a shot), and inexpensive (about $30 for a five-day course). The most common side effects are headaches, hot flashes, mood changes, bloating, and breast tenderness, but most women have few or no side effects. An ultrasound may be done during the first cycle to check the response and adjust the dose if necessary. Usually treatment is limited to six cycles; if clomiphene citrate hasn't worked by then it's unlikely that it's going to.

One problem with clomiphene citrate can limit its effectiveness: in some women it causes changes in the cervical mucus and the lining of the uterus that make it harder to conceive. This can be affected by the dosage you are taking, so increasing your dose is not necessarily the answer when clomiphene doesn't work right away.

Sometimes metformin is added to clomiphene citrate to get better results. Recent studies have shown that your chance of getting pregnant does not increase when metformin is used with clomiphene. However, this combination is recommended as part of fertility treatment if you have glucose intolerance. And you should continue taking it if it is a component of your overall PCOS management plan.

Clomiphene does not increase the risk of birth defects or pregnancy complications. The chance of having twins is much higher, though, and if you do get pregnant with twins your risk

## What Nurses Know...

*You may hear that taking guaifenesin (Robitussin) will improve the cervical mucus. Although this is harmless, there is no real evidence to show that it works. You can find all kinds of remedies for this problem on the Internet, but before you spend your money or risk taking something that may interfere with your efforts to get pregnant talk to your fertility specialist.*

of going into premature labor increases dramatically. You are no more likely to get pregnant with triplets than someone not taking clomiphene.

Concerns have been raised that taking clomiphene citrate increases the risk of ovarian cancer. Recent studies have found this not to be the case with the doses and length of treatment used for fertility treatments.

If you are over 35 years of age or are overweight your fertility specialist may advise you to skip Clomid and go right to step 2, gonadotropins.

**Step 2: Injectable Gonadotropins.** If you have no success with clomiphene citrate the next step is injectable gonadotropins. The principal gonadotropins are FSH and LH, two hormones secreted during the menstrual cycle that stimulate the development of follicles in the ovary and the release of an egg each month. There are two forms of injectable gonadotropins: human menopausal gonadotropin (hMG), natural products made from purified FSH and LH taken from the urine of postmenopausal women (hence their name),and synthetic products. Most natural products contain a combination of FSH and LH (Pergonal, Repronex, Humegon, Menopur), but some have had most or all of the LH removed (Bravelle, Fertinex). Synthetic products include Gonal-F and Follistim and contain only synthesized FSH.

Gonadotropins are given by injection once or twice daily. Most shots are given with a very small needle as subcutaneous injections into the tissue just below the skin, usually on the abdomen or upper thigh. Subcutaneous injections are almost painless, and most women learn to self-inject without any difficulty. Some medications, such as Pergonal and Humegon, must be given via an intramuscular injection into a large muscle, usually in the buttock, with a longer needle. Intramuscular injections hurt a little, and it is usually easier if someone else—your partner, for example—learns to give these to you.

Some women on gonadotropins experience side effects similar to those with clomiphene.

## What Nurses Know . . .

*Do not be put off by the thought of giving yourself injections. Children with diabetes usually start giving themselves insulin injections when they are only 10 years old. You can do it.*

The biggest risks with gonadotropin therapy are ovarian hyperstimulation syndrome (OHSS) and multiple births. Both result from the overstimulation of the ovaries and maturation of multiple follicles. In OHSS the ovaries become swollen and painful. When the condition is severe fluid can leak out of the ovaries into the chest and abdomen. About 10 to 25 percent of women who take gonadotropins experience a mild form of OHSS that gets better on its own after about a week. However, about 2 percent of women develop the more serious form. There is some evidence that women with PCOS have a slightly increased risk of OHSS when taking gonadotropins.

Multiple births are frequent in women who take gonadotropins for fertility. In a natural monthly cycle the level of FSH increases and then decreases, allowing only one follicle to develop to full maturity and only one egg to be released. When FSH levels don't decrease, multiple follicles may reach full maturity, multiple eggs may be released, and you can end up with twins or triplets or more. Gonadotropins are usually administered in a step-up approach to try to prevent this—starting with the minimum dose and increasing it as needed depending on follicle response. This way the dose and duration needed to achieve follicle maturation are minimized. Since this approach became standard the incidence of OHSS and multiple pregnancy has decreased.

During therapy you will be closely monitored with ultrasounds and blood tests to determine when the follicles are mature and you are ready to ovulate. This usually takes 7 to 14 days. At that time you will receive an injection of human chorionic gonadotropin (hCG; Profasi, Pregnyl, Novarel, Ovidrel), which triggers the release of the egg from the follicle. You will be instructed to have intercourse on the day you receive hCG and every other day for about a week.

Your fertility specialist may recommend intrauterine insemination (IUI) along with gonadotropin therapy, either with the first round of gonadotropin injections or if you have not conceived after two or three rounds. A small catheter is inserted through the cervix into the uterus, and sperm is placed directly into the uterus. The procedure takes only a few minutes, and the experience is similar to having a Pap smear. You can return to your normal activities immediately after the procedure. IUI overcomes problems associated with low sperm count or motility and with cervical mucus that is hostile to sperm. It is performed about 36 hours after the hCG injection. Timing is everything, so make sure you administer your injections on time and allow extra time to arrive for the procedure on schedule.

**Step 3: In Vitro Fertilization.**   The final option is in vitro fertilization. Eggs are removed from your ovary, fertilized outside of your body (usually in a Petri dish), and then, after a few days of cell division, transferred into the uterus. In women with PCOS the problem with conception is related to problems with ovulation, so in vitro fertilization is not the first-line treatment. However, it can increase the chance of successful egg fertilization when other methods have failed.

The procedure is similar to IUI until the hCG is injected, though higher doses of gonadotropins are used so that more than one egg matures. At the point at which insemination would take place in IUI, eggs are instead retrieved from your ovary. This procedure is performed under sedation. With ultrasound guidance, a needle is inserted through the vagina into the ovary, and fluid is collected from the mature follicles. This fluid, which contains the eggs, is taken to the lab and placed in an incubator. Sperm is added to fertilize the eggs, and they are allowed to develop for three to five days. You then return to the clinic, and the fertilized eggs (now called embryos) are placed into your uterus using a similar procedure to sperm placement in IUI. After a day of rest you can return to your normal activities.

There is a risk of OHSS with in vitro fertilization. There is also the chance of multiple births, but you can control this by choosing to have just one embryo implanted. Often couples choose to have more than one embryo transferred to increase the chance of success, and this makes a multiple pregnancy more likely.

In vitro fertilization is very expensive. One cycle can cost from $15,000 to $25,000 total. The success rate is the same for women with PCOS as it is for women without PCOS, about 35 percent.

## EMOTIONS

Infertility is devastating for many women. It can cause depression and anxiety and feelings of stigma and isolation. Parents wait for you to make them grandparents. One after another, people in your peer group announce they're expecting. It seems like everyone around you is pregnant or reveling in new parenthood. Even well-meaning friends don't really understand what you're going through, and advice is often misguided or even hurtful. Being told to relax, not to try so hard, that it will just happen, is no help at all.

Fertility treatments are stressful. The uncertainty, the constant monitoring and checking, and the swings between hope and disappointment can leave you feeling as if you're on an emotional roller coaster. Consider counseling to help you through the tough times.

Infertility puts a lot of stress on your relationship with your husband or partner. It can create feelings of inadequacy, failure, anger, and guilt in one or both of you. Having to schedule sex may take some, or all, of the intimacy and fun out of it. However, there are things you can do to support each other and keep your relationship healthy:

• First, keep talking–about infertility and about everything else.

- Take out the paper on which you wrote down your feelings and decisions early on and look at it together periodically.
- Keep sex exciting, spontaneous, and fun. Flirt with each other. Nurture intimacy.
- Infertility will become an obsession if you let it. Don't let it. Plan fun activities. Vacation. Get involved together in a cause, a sport—anything that has nothing to do with infertility.
- Don't put your life on hold. Make plans for the future. You can always revise them if you become pregnant.

Many couples find that their struggles strengthen their bond and deepen their love. Remember: having children was not why you chose to be together. You are together because you love each other and being together makes your lives richer. Not having children shouldn't change that.

## Adoption

Families happen in all kinds of ways. Adoption is an option that most people don't consider until all other options have been

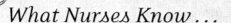

## *What Nurses Know...*

*Talking to family members and close friends about what you're going through can be helpful, but they may need to be educated before they can really be supportive. You may want to give them a book or article about infertility or refer them to a Web site. Sometimes emotion-laden and sensitive information is easier to take in and has more credibility when people hear it from an "expert" or a third party than when they hear it from someone they are attached to—especially when they also have an investment in the subject, as people who care for you do.*

exhausted, but for some it is the method of choice for creating a family. Talk to adoptive parents and you will find their depth of love and connection to their children are no different from those of birth parents. And neither is the amount of joy they find in being a parent.

That doesn't mean adoption is for everyone. And there is nothing wrong with deciding you don't want to adopt. Parenthood is a personal decision that comes from a place so deep that even you may not be sure of the reasons behind it. You don't owe anyone an explanation of your choices. People who have not experienced infertility won't really understand them anyway.

As you go through all the difficulties of fertility treatments, though, it may be helpful to take some time to look into adoption whether or not you are considering it at present. Knowing there is this other option—that no matter what the outcome of the fertility treatments you can still choose to be a parent—may help sustain you. Talk to adoptive parents. Read what adoptive parents have written. You may find that adoption is not your "last hope" but a real choice among many. Or you may decide that it is not for you, after all.

Either way, if fertility treatments are unsuccessful, it is important that you allow yourself time to grieve the loss of the possibility of experiencing pregnancy and childbirth. Although adoption may bring you the joy of finally having the child you want, it also means you are letting go of the biological child you had hoped for.

## Resources

### American Society for Reproductive Medicine

This organization of reproductive health professionals offers fact sheets, booklets, and information on current clinical trials in the Patient section. It also provides a list of affiliated doctors in a number of related specialty areas.

www.asrm.org/

### American Fertility Association

This nonprofit organization is committed to infertility prevention and helping those trying to build a family. It offers guidance and resources on treatment and reproductive health, as well as a database of reproductive professionals and an on-line community.

www.theafa.org/

### Adoptive Families

Online version of the *Adoptive Families* magazine, this site offers comprehensive information about adoption as well as personal stories of adoptees and adoptive parents and family members.

www.adoptivefam.org/

### Resolve

This site, a resource of the National Infertility Association, offers support and information to women and men struggling with infertility. It offers in-depth information on infertility as well as an online community.

www.resolve.org/

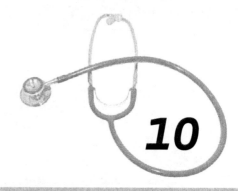

# Looking Ahead

*I'd like to know what's being done about PCOS! People need to pay more attention. There needs to be more research. Doctors need to learn more about it. If I'd had more information or a doctor who knew what was going on ten years ago, maybe I wouldn't have had to struggle so much. Maybe things would be different today.*   STEPHANIE

*There needs to more help, more information. You're constantly dealing with the weight and psychological stuff, and no one really understands. Not even most doctors. You can tell by the comments you hear. I guess that's the biggest things. Everything else is fixable.*   AMY

Most people don't understand PCOS. If they've even heard of it they think it's simply a fertility problem or those heavy women with hair on their chins. Even health care providers often lack information or fail to take your symptoms seriously. Things are beginning to change. More and more people—both health care professionals and the general public—are becoming aware of PCOS and its true scope. We're starting to see more about PCOS in magazines and on Web sites. It is being talked about at medical conferences and written about in professional journals.

A lot of scientific research on PCOS is going on right now. Dozens of studies have been published in medical journals in the past two months alone. Research is beginning to unlock the complex biological processes involved in PCOS. Understanding these processes will lead to better treatment—treatment that will not just improve symptoms but correct the underlying problem.

Recent studies have tried to answer questions on all aspects of PCOS. What is the best approach to weight loss for women with PCOS? What happens if certain medications are used together or at different doses? What behavioral changes are effective? What is the best way to manage infertility in women with PCOS when Clomid doesn't work? Which genes are involved in PCOS? What about the risk of cancer? Or heart disease? What is the relationship between insulin resistance and androgens? Are there ways to predict the chance of getting pregnant?

So new knowledge and better understanding are coming. In the meantime, you now have the knowledge required to be your own best advocate. Start by getting the support you need. Educate the people you care about and who care about you. Give them this book or articles on PCOS to read. E-mail them a link to one of the Web sites in the resource list at the end of this chapter.

Advocate for the best, most up-to-date treatment available. Partner with your health care provider. Talk over options for managing your symptoms. Ask questions. And keep asking until you understand the what, how, and why of every answer.

Living with any chronic condition is difficult, especially when the condition has the far-reaching effects that PCOS has. So be kind to yourself along the way. It isn't easy to make the lifestyle changes the condition demands of you. But be persistent about trying. Keep moving forward.

Remember: you manage PCOS; it doesn't manage you.

## Resources

### Center for Young Women's Health

Web site with extensive information for teenage girls. Conducts periodic online chats for girls with PCOS moderated by nurses, physicians, and nutritionists.

www.youngwomenshealth.org/chat.html

### Hormone Foundation

Web site with information on hormone-related diseases and conditions and patient resources.

www.hormone.org/

### PCOSupport

Web site of the Polycystic Ovarian Syndrome Association, a volunteer, grass-roots, nonprofit organization dedicated to serving women with PCOS. Publishes a weekly newsletter online.

www.pcosupport.org/

### Womenshealth.gov

Federal government Web site with information about PCOS, including a printer-friendly version.

www.womenshealth.gov/faq/polycystic-ovary-syndrome.cfm

# Sample History Form

Date of Birth: _____

Ever sexually active: ☐ Yes ☐ No

Currently sexually active: ☐ Yes ☐ No

## GENERAL

Appetite: _____

Fatigue: _____

## MENSTRUAL HISTORY

Age at onset of menses: _____

Last menstrual period: _____

Frequency of your menstrual periods: _____

Flow: ☐ Heavy ☐ Moderate ☐ Light

Presence of clots: _____

Episodes of abnormal vaginal bleeding: _____

Pain and cramping: _____

## PREGNANCY HISTORY

Time trying to conceive: _____

Number of pregnancies: _____

Number of pregnancies to term: _____

Number of live births: _____

Gestational diabetes: _____

Pregnancy-induced hypertension: _____

Birth control methods used: _____

## WEIGHT

Current weight: _____

Have you had trouble maintaining your ideal body weight?

_____

Are you currently on a diet? _____

Have you had unintentional weight gain or loss? _____

Do you regularly limit how much you eat or how much of certain
types of food you eat? _____

## SKIN

Do you have problems with moderate to severe acne?

      ☐ Yes    ☐ No

If Yes, continue.

When did you first notice problems with acne?_____

_____

Is the acne worse at certain times of the month?_____

_____

Is there anything that worsens the acne?_____

_____

Is there anything that improves the acne? _____

_____

How have you tried to manage it?_____

_____

Were attempts to manage it successful?_____

_____

Discoloration, especially around the neck area   ☐ Yes   ☐ No

## HIRSUTISM

Presence of facial hair              ☐ Yes   ☐ No

Presence of excessive body hair   ☐ Yes   ☐ No

If Yes, continue.

When did you first notice it? _____

How have you tried to manage it?_____

_____

Were attempts to manage it successful?_____

_____

## MALE-PATTERN BALDNESS

Do you have signs of thinning hair or a receding hair line?

      ☐ Yes    ☐ No

If Yes, continue.

When did you first notice it? _____

How have you tried to manage it?_____

_____

Were attempts to manage it successful?_____

_____

## CARDIOVASCULAR
Cholesterol levels: _____

Blood Pressure: _____

## OBSTRUCTIVE SLEEP APNEA
Snoring: _____

Frequent wakening at night: _____

Headaches when you wake up: _____

Daytime sleepiness: _____

## PSYCHOLOGICAL
Depression:   ☐ Yes   ☐ No

Anxiety:   ☐ Yes   ☐ No

## MEDICATIONS
Name: _____

Dose and frequency: _____

When on it and for how long: _____

Effectiveness: _____

Side Effects: _____

## DIAGNOSTIC TESTS DONE (DATES AND RESULTS)
Pelvic ultrasound: _____

Other radiographic tests: _____

Laparoscopy: _____

Endometrial Biopsy: _____

Blood Work (especially hormone levels, cholesterol, glucose tests):

_____

## FAMILY HISTORY
Anyone else in your immediate family with any of the following:

Problems with conceiving or childbirth          ☐ Yes   ☐ No

Menstrual irregularities                                   ☐ Yes   ☐ No

Hirsutism, male-pattern baldness, or moderate to severe acne

                                                                       ☐ Yes   ☐ No

Obesity                                                             ☐ Yes   ☐ No

Diabetes                                                           ☐ Yes   ☐ No

Cardiovascular Disease                                  ☐ Yes   ☐ No

# Glossary

*Note: Definitions listed here cover use of the word in the context of PCOS. Some of these words have additional meanings in other contexts. For complete definitions refer to a general or medical dictionary.*

**Acanthosis nigricans**–brown or black velvety discoloration of the skin usually seen in skin folds, especially around the neck and axilla; most commonly caused by insulin resistance.

**Amenorrhea**–absence of menstrual cycles.

**Androgen**–any substance that produces or stimulates male characteristics; testosterone is the primary androgen.

**Anovulation**–absence of ovulation.

**Apnea**–temporary period of no breathing.

**Arrhythmia**–irregular heart beat.

**Atherosclerosis**–localized lipid-containing plaque in the walls of the blood vessels.

**Autosomal dominant disorder**–only one copy of an abnormal gene is required for a disorder to be inherited.

**BMI (body mass index)**–calculation of body fatness based on the relationship between a person's height and weight.

**Calcification**–deposits of calcium.

**Cerebrovascular**–pertaining to the blood vessels in the brain.

**Comedone**–sebaceous gland plugged with dried sebum; blackheads and whiteheads.

**Corpus luteum**–temporary component of the ovary that develops from the follicle after ovulation; secretes estrogen and progesterone; important in proliferation and shedding of the endometrium during the menstrual cycle.

**Cutaneous**–pertaining to the skin, including the hair.

**Differential diagnosis**–a process for distinguishing among diseases, conditions, and syndromes with similar symptoms when trying to make a diagnosis.

**Diuretic**–drug or natural substance that increases the output of urine.

**Electrocoagulation**–use of high-frequency electric current that generates heat to destroy tissue.

**Endocrine system**–glands that secrete hormones.

**Endocrinologist**–physician who specializes in hormonal diseases, including PCOS, diabetes, and thyroid disease.

**Endometrium**–lining of the uterus; proliferates and then sheds cyclically under the influence of hormones during the menstrual cycle.

**Etiology**–cause of a disease, condition, or syndrome.

**Follicle-stimulating hormone (FSH)**–hormone secreted by the pituitary gland that stimulates the maturation of ovarian follicles.

**Genetic marker**–identifiable gene with a known chromosome location.

**Gestational diabetes**–high blood sugar during pregnancy in women who did not have diabetes before the pregnancy.

**Glucocorticoid**–steroid hormone originating in the adrenal gland that is involved in carbohydrate metabolism and the immune system.

**Gonadotropin**–hormone that stimulates the sex glands, either the ovaries or testes.

**Gonadotropin-releasing hormone (GnRH)**–hormone secreted by the hypothalamus that stimulates the production and release of luteinizing hormone and follicle-stimulating hormone from the pituitary gland.

**Heterogeneous**–composed of multiple types, characteristics, or elements.

**Hirsutism**–excessive growth of hair or growth of hair in unusual places, such as facial hair in women.

**Homogeneous**–composed of like or uniform types, characteristics, or elements.

**Hyperandrogenemia**–higher than normal levels of androgens in the blood.

**Hyperandrogenism**–excessive secretion of androgens, usually referring to the clinical signs such as hirsutism and virilism.

**Hyperinsulinemia**–excessive concentration of insulin in the blood.

**Hyperplasia**–overgrowth of cells and tissue.

**Hypertension**–high blood pressure; usually defined as systolic pressure (top number) equal to or greater than 140 and diastolic pressure (lower number) equal to or greater than 90.

**Idiopathic**–disease, condition, or disorder that has no known cause.

**Intramuscular**–into the muscle.

**Jaundice**–yellowing of the skin, eyes, and mucous membranes related to too much bilirubin in the blood; can be due to liver, pancreas, or gallbladder disease or to excess destruction of red blood cells.

**Lactation**–secretion of milk from mammary glands; breast-feeding.

**Lipids**–fat substances in the blood (cholesterol, triglycerides).

**Luteinizing hormone (LH)**–a hormone secreted by the pituitary gland that has a role in the maturation of ovarian follicles and triggers ovulation.

**Macronutrients**–carbohydrate, protein, and fat; nutrients that the body uses in large quantities.

**Malaise**–generalized feeling of discomfort or feeling unwell.

**Metabolic**–pertaining to the chemical activity in the body.

**Oligo-ovulation**–infrequent ovulation.

**Ovulation**–the release of an ovum (egg) from a mature ovarian follicle.

**Pathological**–due to disease; diseased.

**Polycystic**–having many cysts.

**Sebum**–oily, fatty substance secreted by sebaceous glands.

**Subcutaneous**–under the skin.

**Virilization**–signs of masculinization in a female.

# Index